# What They Didn't Teach You at Medical School

Alan V. Parbhoo

# What They Didn't Teach You at Medical School

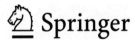 Springer

Alan V. Parbhoo
MBBS (London), Bsc (Hons.), MRCS (England)
St Bartholmew's and Royal London Hospitals NHS Trust
London, UK

British Library Cataloguing in Publication Data
A catalogue record for this book is available from the British Library

Library of Congress Control Number: 2006935875

ISBN-10: 1-84628-461-9          e-ISBN-10: 1-84628-733-2
ISBN-13: 978-1-84628-461-8      e-ISBN-13: 978-1-84628-733-6

Printed on acid-free paper

9 8 7 6 5 4 3 2 1

Springer Science+Business Media
springer.com

# Contents

# Introduction

When I graduated I started work in a 950-plus bed then district general hospital, which subsequently became the flagship teaching hospital of the UK, that is the first private funding initiative hospital to be built. Not only was it chaotic to move an entire hospital from one building to another several miles down the road, but I was thrown in at the deep end clinically, to say the least. In my second week as a house officer I was scheduled to do nights, which meant looking after all the medical in-patients alone. In cases of emergency I could call the medical senior house officer (SHO) from the medical assessment unit. It was a case of sink or swim and swim hard I did. *The Hands-on Guide for House Officers*[1] and the *Oxford Handbook of Clinical Medicine*[2] (Cheese and Onion) became my best friends, but I could not help but notice that there were certain things in the day-to-day tasks that I had not learnt at medical school and were not in the books. There are some skills that medical students are expected to learn by 'osmosis' while on placement and under the guidance of junior doctors. These skills are never officially taught or examined in medical school. They are, however, a fundamental part of being a safe, good and efficient doctor.

I found that as a junior theoretically simple tasks when put into practice take a long time and are frustrating to organise and complete. When I was a pre-registration house officer (PRHO) there were normally other staff around that I could ask, but they always seemed so busy and I wanted a guide on hand. When I asked around, my colleagues and I were all in the same boat. We had the knowledge (the map) and we thought we knew how to be doctors (we had been to medical school and therefore could read a map), but there was a missing link (the map was in a different language)!

---

[1] Donald A, Stein M. *The Hands-on Guide for House Officers*, 2nd edn. Oxford: Blackwell; 2002.
[2] Longmore M, Wilkinson I, Torok E. *Oxford Handbook of Clinical Medicine*, 5th edn. Oxford: Oxford University Press; 2002.

This book is meant to help you read the map in front of you – to unlock your potential and improve your performance. To scythe down the amount of time it takes you to do things. It is meant to fill in the gaps where medical school and clinical guides have stopped. This book is designed to give you the information you need to organise your firm so you can hit the ground running. It is not intended as a clinical survival guide, but more how to help you get ahead in medicine and how to keep on track and develop a career path.

This guide will teach you how to get on with others in the workplace and learn how to pass patient information to them appropriately and concisely, earning you respect and giving you skill.

This book is not just for final year medical students and PRHOs. It covers all the information you need to begin to carve out a career and will provide much information required by SHOs alike to get you a step ahead of the rest of the crowd at each point in your career pathway.

Just to put you in the picture …

In 2003, 13 583 students applied to study medicine in the UK, but only 7824 of those were accepted.[3] Most know that there is a shortfall in the number of doctors required to meet the growing needs of the National Health Service and it is estimated that, by 2005, there will be 7300 medical school places in England alone to meet the demand.[4] With the size of medical school class years increasing, it is likely that the transfer of 'hand me down' information and skills learnt piecemeal from doctors while on placements will decrease. This book is therefore designed to help fill in the political, medical, surgical, philosophical and administrative gaps that are not fulfilled by the curriculum at medical school.

The book includes 'golden rules' or important points to remember – ignore these at your peril…! – and case examples, both of which are given as displayed extracts.

This book is designed to be dipped into or read front to back, whichever is your preference. It makes good bedtime reading as it is not too strenuous and hopefully will make you smile.

I have tried as much as possible to write about what I feel is important and not taught in medical schools, but if I have covered things you already know then I apologise. However, if there are items I have not covered, then I ask you to drop me an e-mail and let me know your thoughts.

PLEASE NOTE: I have used the terms pre-registration house officer (PRHO) and senior house officer (SHO) in this book. These are being replaced by FY1 and FY2 respectively, but I have stuck to traditional terms to avoid confusion.

---

[3] Thanks to Christine Vera-Cruz at the University and Colleges Application Service.
[4] Making the medical school grade. *The Sunday Times* 14 September 2003.

# Acknowledgements

I would like to thank Professor Nick Cheshire, who is the first consultant I have worked with, who has taken the time to see my potential and treat me as an equal rather than a subordinate. He prompted me to collect my thoughts and opinions on medical student teaching and write this book. I know he thought that, once I had left his employ, that the idea would have been laid to rest. I was pleased to surprise him when I returned from a nine-month honeymoon with the first draft!

I also thank my beautiful wife Teja who has encouraged me to speak my mind when writing this book. As a physiotherapist she has been able to give me valuable insight into the roles and responsibilities that go with her job.

My parents, who foolishly brought me into this world (little did they know what they were getting themselves into), have given me the integrity to stand up for my beliefs and be eternally vigilant when it comes to caring for others. My father in particular inspired me to become a doctor and has given me an incredible gift, continued support and keen surgical hands.

Sincere thanks are due to Mr Boyd Goldie who put me in touch with John Harrison, a man who has taken a leap of faith by taking on this book where other publishers thought the content too 'competitive' with their other products.

To you, the reader for buying this text – I hope you find it useful and I ask you to pass the knowledge imparted to you to your peers and juniors.

There are many doctors and nurses who have kindly offered nuggets of information or taken the time to read sections of this book and appraise them. In particular I would like to thank Sameer Khurjekar, Kathryn Powrie, Duncan Powrie and Ashok Menon.

Last and by no means least, a great deal of thanks go to a man with far more talent than he would have you believe – a legendary problem solver at the Royal Free, artist and all-round nice guy, Bernie Cousins.

# 1

# A Brief History of the National Health Service

The National Health Service (NHS) is the largest organisation in the UK and the biggest employer in Europe. It took decades before any consensus between doctors and politicians could be made as to how it should be set up and what its requirements were. Before the Second World War there was a large disparity between those receiving good medical care and those who were not. There was a disparity between access to hospitals, specialist doctors and general community medicine. Before 1943 the only free medical care available was in the event of an emergency and only in certain hospitals at that, for example the Royal Free Hospital (hence the term 'free').

By 1943, after several years of war, the 'idea of free and comprehensive service for all'[1] was already being discussed as there were strong feelings between both doctors and politicians in the light of how the war had affected and injured rich and poor alike.

Sir William Beveridge was commissioned by the government to write a report on the state of the nation. This report on future social insurance was published in 1942 and laid out five areas that needed improvement if the nation was to survive: want, disease, ignorance, squalor and idleness.[2]

In 1944 the Goodenough Report was produced to outline the provision of medical services versus the provision of medical education. One could not exist without the other. It was decided shortly thereafter that there should be an even distribution of medical schools throughout the country.

The first person really to organise unity between the politicians and the medical profession was Aneurin Bevan, the Health Minister in 1946. He created and empowered

---

[1] Ministry of Health. *Report of the Office Committee on the 'Demobilisation' of the Emergency Hospital Scheme.* London: Ministry of Health; 1943.

[2] Parliament (Chairman: Sir William Beveridge). *Report on Social and Insurance and Allied Services*, Cmd 6040. London: HMSO; 1942.

the NHS Act of 1946 to establish 'a comprehensive health service to secure the improvement in the physical and mental health of the people … and the prevention, diagnosis and treatment of illness'. The act was set out to regionalise all services to include the previously separated universities, voluntary hospitals, private hospitals and general practices in order to generate a united health service.

It took several years to establish these health regions and to organise services and on 5 July 1948 the new NHS began.

# 2

# Modern National Health Service Trusts

Some of you may have already heard of the National Health Service (NHS) Modernisation Agency. This grand-sounding group of people have been given the cumbersome task of dragging the NHS into the twenty-first century and beyond (not quite like Buzz Lightyear, but similar). The NHS, as you are aware, is segregated into hundreds if not thousands of trusts throughout the country, each of which has mountains of policies. In true governmental style these policies are the living personification of bureaucracy and often have little or no clinical reasoning. Those that have been implemented through clinical reasoning are out of date. Therefore, it will take Buzz or some other space age technique to sort all the mess out and improve patient care.

The task of the NHS Modernisation Agency is an unenviable one, but they have come up with ten so-called and, I quote, 'high impact changes that organisations … can adopt to make significant, measurable improvements in … care'[1] (Table 2.1). The aim of this is to reduce waiting times and improve the accuracy of treatment by changing the way we do things. A more streamlined approach to care, with better organisation, is what is needed: managing patient admissions and discharges across the country in order to reduce the variation, increasing day case surgery and procedures in order to decrease the in-patient waiting list, faster and more streamlined investigation of acute and chronic disease, etc.

Having read the document I am still not sure what a care bundle approach is other than it comes from our friends across the Atlantic and seems to be set by doctors and is evidence based, which must be a good thing.

In order to consider the NHS you must understand its sheer scale and stand in awe at how good it really is. We do actually have one of the best health services in the

---

[1] NHS Modernisation Agency. *10 High Impact Changes for Service Improvement and Delivery: A Guide for NHS Leaders.* 2004.

---

**Table 2.1** The ten high-impact changes

---

Treat day surgery as the norm for elective surgery
Improve access to key diagnostic tests
Manage variation in patient discharge
Manage variation in patient admission
Avoid unnecessary follow-ups
Increase the reliability of performing therapeutic interventions through a care
  bundle approach
Apply a systematic approach to care for people with long-term conditions
Improve patient access by reducing the number of queues
Optimise patient flow using process templates
Redesign and extend roles

---

world, despite what you read or see in the news. It is easy to become disillusioned in the NHS and think that it does not work or that the care could be much better.

The question is how many hospitals do you think there are in the UK, how many employees are there and how many patients are treated a year? Hundreds, thousands and millions, respectively?… What about the cost of running even one single NHS trust? Hundreds of thousands, millions or billions of pounds?

There are 1.28 million NHS employees in the UK, but only half of these are medical personnel (doctors, nurses, therapists, etc.).[2] One would assume therefore that there are an awful lot of managers and clerical staff out there.

In London alone there are 27 NHS hospital trusts plus the London Ambulance Service NHS trust. The budget for an average-sized district general hospital (DGH) with university hospital status (that is a DGH that accepts medical students on placement, but has no academic departments or research programmes like a true teaching hospital) is £150 million per year.[3] Multiply by 28 and add the extra cost of the teaching hospitals and the budget for London is at the very least £4.5 billion. That is an awful lot of national insurance contributions!

When the Electronic Patient Record (EPR) is fully operational in 2010 the NHS will have the largest computer system in the world. The EPR is a phenomenal undertaking and will be truly spectacular when running. It is costing billions of pounds to install the millions of miles of secure broadband cabling up and down the country to connect every hospital and general practice to the system. Not to mention the provision of new computers for every workstation and smart cards that will allow swipe access to the system for every member of staff. The 'choose and book' system is part of the EPR and you will have no doubt have seen it in the news.

---

[2] Health managers' pay soars (pity about the nurses). *Daily Mail* 16 February 2005.
[3] Based on Whipps Cross University Hospital NHS trust.

# 3

# Applying for Pre-registration House Officer Posts

## The Pre-registration House Officer Is in Danger of Extinction... and What Will Replace It?

There has unfortunately been a large change in junior doctor training over the last few years initially with the introduction of the European Working Time Directive (EWTD) and more recently with Modernising Medical Careers (MMC). The pre-registration house officer (PRHO) is now an endangered species. No longer will those who are graduating become PRHOs and then Senior House Officers (SHOs). You will now become 'Foundation Trainees'.

There has been a gradual shift across the country to replace traditional training with a new 'updated' training scheme to fast-track newly qualified doctors through the system to become more senior more quickly than in the old system. Everyone knows that the number of years it takes to train to become a consultant is less than it was 10 or even 5 years ago. However, adding the EWTD on to this means that we work less hours. Less hours per day for less years results in less skilled and less experienced doctors which will result in poorer patient care.

Patients complain that all too often, they do not meet their consultant in the outpatient clinic but see a junior member of the team. This is understandable and just one of the ways that patient's are unhappy about the service that is being provided. The public has become more demanding of the NHS over the past decade and as a profession we have failed to provide enough patient education to explain why junior doctors are such a fundamental part of the team. At the end of the day, today's junior doctors will be tomorrow's consultants, and we need to see as many patients as possible to gain the experience required to fulfil a consultant role.

It is this fundamental naivety between the public and those that manage the National Health Service which has catalysed the change in junior doctor training.

The medical side of the NHS is now to become a consultant-led service as per the demands of the public. This will mean an increase in the number of consultant posts available but the introduction of weekend and evening NHS work, resident on-call and shift work for consultants. This is part of the existing 'new' consultant contract and fears of what are to come. The shift to increasing the number of consultants in the NHS is a wolf in sheep's clothing. The public want a higher standard of care but what they may get is the opposite. Doctors want better training but what we are currently getting is the opposite. The removal of the PRHO is yet another step in modernising training and many junior and senior doctors have grave reservations about the new Foundation Scheme. However, not everything about modernising medical careers (MMC) is bad and certainly the quality of life Foundation Trainees will have is far greater than their predecessors. Certain parts of the Foundation syllabus are to be commended and the overall doctor which it is trying to create is one who has an overall understanding of patient centred care, good communication, and a keen eye to spot a sick patient and prevent clinical incidents. I agree that this can only be a good thing but at what expense – knowledge and experience? Perhaps….

## Foundation Schemes

The Foundation Scheme is a two-year programme divided into an F1 year (year 1 which is approximately equivalent to current PRHO training) and an F2 year (which is equated to year 1 of an SHO).

The Foundation programme has been designed to produce 'demonstrably competent doctors who are skilled at communicating and working as effective members of a team'.[1] The last time I checked, it was important for a doctor to have sound understanding of the functioning (anatomy, physiology and biochemistry) and malfunctioning (pathology) of the human body as well as a basic capacity to be an effective communicator and team player. When I was at medical school it was the task of the interview panel to decide whether you were skilled in the latter two. I should state that I do not think that those exiting the Foundation Scheme will be as poorly trained as some of my senior colleagues fear. However, despite major concerns regarding purely 'academic' teaching, there are aspects of the Foundation Programme which deserve credit. The core areas of assessment are outlined in the *Curriculum for the foundation years in postgraduate education and training*. The structure examines three

---

[1] Department of Health. *Modernising Medical Careers*. 2003. The Response of the 4 UK Health Ministers to the Consultation on Unfinished Business: proposals for the reform of the SHO grade. Department of Health, London.

areas: knowledge, attitudes and skills.[2] The subjects of assessment are broad and while there is no mention of despite what a lot of us think is a conflict of interests, this new system began being phased in during 2004 and is due to replace the old system completely by 2007.

The F1 year will consist of three four-month posts in medicine, surgery and one other specialty. The F2 year is split into three four-month placements including accident and emergency (A&E) followed by two blocks of either surgical or medical specialities. Alternatively the year is split into four three-month placements and this depends on which area of the country you apply to. Other specialties may be taken in addition to medicine and surgery, but these have not been finalised. However, these are reported to include A&E, critical care, general practice, obstetrics and gynaecology, paediatrics, pathology and psychiatry.[3]

As no fixed programme of training has been finalised for those exiting the F2 year we still do not know how the training or postgraduate examinations of the Royal Colleges will be organised. It is thought (or hoped) that a scheme will be finalised by 2006, but until then we will have to rely on our imagination (Figure 3.1).

My advice would be to clerk, examine, investigate and treat as many patients as you possible can in the short training that you will have as this will be the only possible way of gaining experience. I do not wish for you to finish reading this chapter and think that your training will be poor or that I am against change. Far from it, I think that your training will be different and none of us (including you) have any idea just what tomorrow's doctors will be like. I find this of grave concern but we all have to 'accept the things I/we cannot change, the courage to change the things I/we can, and the wisdom to know the difference' [Reinhold Niebuhr]. When I am more senior I may be inclined not to accept, but to change.

## Teaching Hospital or District General Hospital?

Most undergraduates are under the impression that teaching hospitals are the be all and end all when it comes to house jobs. This is not necessarily the case and it depends on what you wish to gain from your house jobs/FY1. Teaching hospitals are big names and, as such, competition is high when you apply. This is not just at the PRHO level. However, they can offer teaching on the latest research and techniques

---

[2] The Foundation Programme Committee of the Academy of Medical Royal Colleges, in co-operation with Modernising Medical Careers in the Departments of Health. *Curriculum for the foundation years in postgraduate education and training.* London: Department of Health; 2005.

[3] *Foundation Programme Pilot Schemes Monitoring Report to the Junior Doctors Committee and the Medical Students Committee.* British Medical Association; 2004 (www.bma.org.uk/ap.nsf/content/fndtnpilotmonitor).

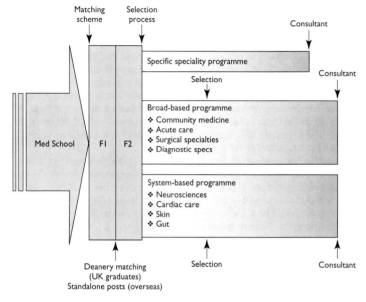

**Figure 3.1** Proposed outline of training (*Student BMJ* 2005; 13: 1–44).

as well as more obscure and complex clinical pathology (as they are often tertiary referral centres, that is they accept referrals from other hospitals. A primary referral is where a patient self-refers to a general practitioner (GP) or A&E department, and secondary referral is where a patient is referred to hospital by a GP). The downside to this is two-fold. You do not see as much 'bread and butter' disease and teaching hospitals attract research and training staff from all over the world. The consequence is that the firm size is often large with perhaps two SHOs, two SpRs and a research fellow and occasionally more. This means that there are many trainees competing to get into clinics and theatre as well as ward-based activities, particularly practical procedures. Consequently, as a PRHO, there is little scope for learning many practical procedures or operative surgery. On the other hand, it is easier to apply for a teaching hospital rotation if you have worked there as a PRHO, so there are pros and cons.

District general hospitals (DGHs), however, are less competitive and offer greater opportunities for seeing 'bread and butter' medical and surgical case presentations as well as the practical procedures that go alongside them. For example, if you saw a patient with suspected meningitis in a DGH you would be expected to perform a supervised lumbar puncture after you had seen a couple (the 'see one, do one, teach one' philosophy is still alive and kicking!). If you were working in a teaching hospital the SHO or SpR would almost certainly perform the lumbar puncture.

Although I have stated that it is marginally easier to get an SHO post in a teaching hospital if you have worked there as a PRHO, there is no reason why anyone should not be able to get a teaching hospital job if they are good enough and are enthusiastic. For example, those who have chalked up a good number of practical skills will be well sought after as an SHO. If you have been involved in audit this will also get you some 'brownie points'.

## Matching Schemes: Job or No Job?

My year was one of the first to have a matching scheme for finding a PRHO post, but it is now the norm. In fact there are now matching schemes for the PRHO, FY1 and FY2 programmes. Each medical school is linked to other hospitals within its geographical region and in theory there should be enough posts for all graduating students. However, in practice this does not always work due to various 'acts of God' for which your medical school or the government cannot possibly take responsibility (heaven forbid if they actually generate a scheme that (1) works and is reliable and (2) is easy to apply for: most schemes seem more complicated than quantum physics).

If you are one of the individuals who ends up without a post or less commonly without two posts then fear not – you are not the only one. I found myself in the situation where I had a post organised for the second half of my house year, but the matching scheme failed to find me my first house post. My medical school were not helpful at giving me any information on how to go about finding a post for the first six months and I know this was not an isolated example. I had a difficult time trying to find out how to apply for jobs, never mind get an interview. I have written this section in the hope that it will reduce your stress levels and also cut down the time it takes you.

Despite previous problems with matching schemes, I have been reliably informed that they are now more efficient and streamlined.

## Finding a Vacant Post

This is easy when you know how and there are three places where jobs are advertised.

1 The *British Medical Journal* classifieds: this is the most popular and you can find it in three ways: on-line at http://www.bmjcareers.com, by subscribing to the

*British Medical Journal* or reading it in your medical school library. The classifieds are published every Friday and contain all jobs listed by speciality and grade. There is an 'ad alert' facility on the website where you can save a search and run it each time you go to the website, for example:

"jobs | hospital appointments | gastroenterology | house officer | London"

The search facility is so good that you can even get it to e-mail you with new postings as soon as they are published. This is an excellent website that is free to use. You do not have to be a member of the British Medical Association to use the service, which is a bonus.

2 www.Doctors.net.uk: this is a website for doctors by doctors and has a lot more than just job advertisements. It also contains sections on medical news, training and an on-line library. Click on the jobs section to access the search facility. At the time of writing this site does not have as many advertisements as the *British Medical Journal*, but it is growing in popularity and will become more useful as time marches on.

3 In-house stop press: this is an advertising scheme run by the human resources or medical staffing department of each hospital. Often the recruitment officer will know about impending post availabilities long before they are advertised. It is the wise who prepare their application beforehand.

## Applying for a Post

Once you have found a post or posts that tickle your fancy you must apply. There is no limit to the number of posts you may apply for, but you will find that each application takes a lot of time and energy so you become selective pretty quickly! All advertisements have a reference code, which is different for every job. Most advertisements will also list a 24-hour answerphone number or e-mail address. All you have to do is leave your name and address along with the job reference on the answerphone and the hospital will send you an application pack (application form, occupational health questionnaire, police check form, details about the hospital, trust and the post). Some advertisements instruct the applicant to simply send a number of curricula vitae (CVs) with a covering letter. Over the last few years medical human resources departments have become digitally aware and allow on-line applications where the forms can be downloaded, filled in and e-mailed back. This is the way forward, but if you file an application this way then telephone to confirm that your application has been received as e-mail is not infallible!

Regardless of what the advertisement specifies, when you send off your application always send a copy of your CV with a covering letter, which should be typed in a standard business format. If possible speak to the PRHO or SHO who is currently doing that job to find out the inside word. It is usually not possible to speak with or meet the consultant organising the interviews until the short-listing is done.

## Interviews

If you are short-listed then congratulations! You will be among the 15–20 candidates short-listed from several hundred others and should be proud to make it this far. Next is to prepare for the interview. You should spend at least a few days doing a bit of research for the big day.

1   Find out if the consultant has published any research recently and make sure that you know about the topic. It can be a useful piece of conversation during or at the end of an interview. When asked if you have any questions you can ask about current research in the department and act interested.
2   Make sure you have spoken to the current PRHO/SHO.
3   Find out some of the history and reputation of the hospital you are applying to.
4   Take particular note of whether the hospital has achieved any major medical landmarks, for example the Royal Free Hospital was the site of the first kidney transplant with immunosuppression.
5   Make sure you have basic knowledge of the speciality you are applying for, as occasionally you may be asked clinical scenario-based questions in the interview. These are to test your pattern of thinking rather than your knowledge, so do not be alarmed.

Finally, there is one golden rule: never attend an interview for a post which you would not be happy to accept if offered on the day. This used to be quite strict but is becoming more relaxed. If you have several interviews on the go it is not unreasonable to state this when offered a job. However, you must give a time frame as to when you will give them an answer. This should be a prompt as possible.

# 4

# Surviving the Pre-registration House Officer Post

## Introduction

The pre-registration house officer (PRHO) post, soon to become the F1 year, is a tough year, there is no doubt about it. However, it should also be a fun and stimulating year as you finally get to put into practice all the things you have learnt at medical school. There is nothing quite like your first pay cheque to put a smile on your face and a load on your liver.

There will be good and bad times ahead, but I hope the sections in this chapter may make it easier for you to look after your patients and do what is required of you. Do not forget that, if you get into difficulties, there are always others around whom you can ask for help. Speak up and you will be surprised to see who comes to your rescue!

## Prioritising the Working Day

This is a topic that newly qualified doctors find particularly difficult. After the often busy and chaotic morning ward round with your consultant or specialist registrar (SpR), how do you know what to do next and in what order. The most obvious statement is to organise all the urgent tasks first, whether that be requesting investigations, performing procedures or referring patients to other teams. However, after the urgent things the list becomes grey. Reassuringly, your skill in prioritisation increases exponentially with the number of posts you have done so that, by the time you are a senior house officer (SHO), you should have it honed (Table 4.1).

## To Take Away Sheets

'To take away' (TTA) or 'to take out' sheets are A4 pieces of paper with triplicate carbon copies on the back that contain a prescription of the drugs a patient is to take

**Table 4.1** How to prioritise tasks

| Time of day | Task to hand |
| --- | --- |
| Immediately post-ward round | Urgent investigation requests[a] |
| | Urgent patient examination |
| | Urgent in-patient referrals |
| Early morning | In-patient investigations to be done within 24 hours |
| | In-patient procedures |
| | In-patient referrals |
| Late morning[b] | Non-urgent in-patient investigation requests |
| | Non-urgent in-patient referrals |
| Afternoon | Out-patient investigation requests |
| | Out-patient referrals |
| Late afternoon[b] | Blood test requests for the following day |
| | Write blood results in notes for today's tests |
| | Go home! |

[a] These should always be discussed with the on-call radiologist or laboratory technicians in order to expedite them.
[b] Do find time in your day to squeeze in a coffee or some toast, but do not expect to get the breaks every two hours as stipulated in the European Work Time Directive!

home with them on discharge from hospital. They have been extended over the years to include a mini discharge summary and follow-up information, which you need to write clearly (usually in capitals) for four reasons.

1 One copy goes with the patient so that if they see their general practitioner (GP) or come back to hospital within a few days of leaving then the GP or accident and emergency (A&E) department SHO knows what has been done to the patient and what the diagnosis was.

2 A copy goes in the patient notes.

3 A copy is posted to the GP on the day of discharge, which provides the GP with brief details of the admission until the discharge summary arrives.

4 The SpR often uses it to assist in writing the official discharge letter. This is posted to the patient's GP and usually this takes about two to four weeks, often much longer. In some trusts it is never written/posted at all. Discharge summaries are usually written some weeks after the patient has been discharged and it is difficult for the SpR or SHO to remember them. The TTA sheet acts as a very useful memory aid and good TTA sheets are greatly appreciated by seniors.

Ideally TTA sheets should be done 24–48 hours before the patient is expected to be discharged. This is because the ward pharmacist has to collect the form and then take it to the pharmacy, which then dispenses the medication. Then the whole lot is brought back to the ward. This sometimes takes a whole day. Medical ward rounds are notoriously slow and TTA sheets can usually be written on the round while the SHO writes in the patient notes. Surgical rounds are a little too short and sweet and TTA sheets are therefore normally written afterwards (note that the rounds are so short you will need to write in the notes after the round). As a house officer you will often have three to five TTA sheets to write per day. It is sensible to prioritise these as there will always be late or unexpected patient discharges and their TTA sheets should be done first.

## Note Keeping

This is one of the arms of clinical governance and it has received a lot of attention over the last few years.

Medico-legally, each piece of paper or document regarding a patient must have the following information on it: patient surname, forename and hospital number. With each entry it is important to have the following clearly written in the notes: date, time, surname of the staff member seeing the patient, position and bleep number. The reason for this is accountability. Each individual should be responsible for his or her own actions and by identifying yourself you are taking that responsibility. More importantly you are documenting the care of that patient.

The nurses may query any instructions or plans that you write in the notes and they may wish to discuss them with you. Finally and by no means least, if you perform a practical procedure, for example a catheterisation, chest drain insertion, etc., it is vital for you to write your name, grade and bleep number. This is because, if there is a complication, the nursing staff will need to inform you so you can attend to the patient. This is also for your own education so you can see if you have made an error and therefore learn from your mistakes.

## Medical Notes and Medical Records

More often than not your consultants and seniors will recount tales of old about long searches for radiographs and patient notes for ward rounds and meetings. Hundred of hours a month are wasted searching for patient notes and their radiographs in preparation for ward rounds and elective patient admissions. Thankfully, with the advent of twenty-first-century information technology into the health service some of us are now 'privileged' to work in hospitals with digital radiology. By 2010 the Electronic Patient Record should be in place making paper notes a thing of the past. Unfortunately, until such times arrive it will still be the task of the PRHO to locate files and films for the consultant or SpR.

This thankless task can be made easier by knowing certain facts about tracking systems within hospitals. The hospital number on a computer system tracks patient notes. The medical records department is a large vault of a department that is usually located in the bowels of the hospital, the basement being the commonest site. All patient notes should be stored in the medical records department unless someone in the hospital is using them. Each consultant or office, department and cleric in the hospital has their own code and when notes are taken from the medical records department it should be recorded on the medical records department computer system, providing they have been booked or 'tracked' to the person who has borrowed them. For example, if a patient attends the chest clinic the notes will be booked out to the clinic under the name of the consultant they are seeing. When the patient has been seen and the clinic letter typed, the notes should then be returned to the medical records department.

When you are asked to get a set of case notes the first thing to do is to ask your consultant's secretary to check where the notes are on the computer system (usually called the Patient Administration System or PAS). If the notes are in the medical records department then the task is easy: go and collect them, but remember to book them out to your consultant. If they are not in the medical records department then see if they have been booked out, when they were and to whom. Get the telephone extension of the person who has booked them out and ask them if they have them, etc.

When notes are not where they should be problems occur and usually it is not possible to find them. In this situation it can take hours and hours to find them often without success. My advice here is to become friends with the ward clerk or your consultant's secretary and persuade them to do the legwork. Ultimately you will have to tell your consultant that you could not fulfil his/her request.

## Radiographs and the Film Library

The X-ray archive or film library serves the same purpose as the medical records department, but for all radiological investigations, for example plain radiographs, computed tomographs and magnetic resonance images.

Not everybody books out films when they borrow them and this is particularly the case when doctors borrow them for meetings. Many senior doctors are in the habit of simply picking up the notes/films and borrowing them without telling anyone.

When you are asked to get a set of films the first thing to do is to telephone the film library and see if the films are there. If they are, then easy: go and collect them, but remember to book them out to your consultant. If they are not in the archive then see if they have been booked out, when they were and to whom. Get the telephone extension of the person who has booked them out and ask them if they have them and so on.

When X-ray images are missing it is sometimes possible to persuade the radiology department to reprint the films if they have a copy on their computer system, but you will have to be very skilled in the art of persuasion or very good at chatting someone up – usually the radiographers!

## Equipment

All PRHOs need certain basic and inexpensive tools of the trade, which they should already have from being a medical student. You will no doubt see and hear newly qualified doctors flouncing around with a brand new set of cardiology guessing tubes (because they cannot train their ear to use a regular stethoscope) or other suchlike expensive equipment. This kind of kit is useful as you become more senior (SHO and SpR level). The equipment that you do need after graduation for your PRHO post is given in Table 4.2.

Most will be glad to know that you do not need a tendon hammer, ophthalmoscope/otoscope or expensive stethoscope. Most specialist equipment will be available on the appropriate wards, for example a tendon hammer on a neurology ward, an otoscope on an ear, nose and throat ward (ENT), etc. If you need to use this equipment, the nursing staff on the respective wards will often lend it to you if you are nice to them.

## Pre-admission Clinics

These are the sole responsibility of the junior doctor on the firm and most often the PRHO. The purpose of these clinics is to assess patients one to two weeks before their elective admission to hospital. Your job is to clerk the patients, that is take a history and examine and perform basic investigations (bloods, electrocardiograph and radiographs) on the patient, to either streamline their admission or make sure they are fit for an elective operation. It is not uncommon for operations to be delayed or cancelled

Table 4.2 The PRHOs toolbox

| Type of equipment | Available from |
| --- | --- |
| Classic stethoscope | Littmann™ |
| Tourniquet | Free from drug representatives |
| Brain | Everyone is born with one, but many PRHOs forget to use it |
| Eyes | The best diagnostic equipment available and free with every birth! |
| Ears | See eyes |
| Common sense | Fundamental for a successful career in medicine: unfortunately, you either have it or you do not and it cannot be bought on E-bay™ |

based on the findings of the PRHO, as the patient may not have been seen in the out-patient department for many months.

These clinics are straightforward and nothing to be feared if you are diligent and thorough. If you have clinic nurses they are usually very experienced, friendly and used to helping newly qualified doctors along the way. Unfortunately, on occasion, these nurses have been the victim of new PRHOs' arrogance and may be a little caustic to start with. If you find them unpleasant, introduce yourself and talk to them. They will soon get to know and like you. If you are lucky you may even get brought cups of tea and biscuits as I used to!

## Out-patient Clinics

Further to the section on clinics (see Chapter 11), as a PRHO you may be asked to attend out-patient clinics. They are run as already outlined, but it is important to be on good terms with the nursing staff as they can be a tremendous source of help both in organising yourself, but also in dealing with awkward or angry patients. As a junior you may well require a chaperone and it is good professional practice to ask for one if your patient is of the opposite sex and of a similar age (this particularly applies to male doctors for obvious reasons). Depending on your consultant, you may be expected to dictate clinic letters (or your consultant may chose to do this after they have seen the patient). There is a particular order and method for this, which differs from team to team and you should ask your seniors to teach you in the first few weeks of the post (you will be provided with a dictaphone, so for the wealthy among you, do not contemplate buying one!). At the end of the clinic you should deliver the tape (available from your consultant's secretary – hint: get it before you go to the clinic) and the patients' notes to the secretary who will type the letters for you to sign a day or two later. Once signed, the letters can be posted to the patients' GPs. Sign them promptly or the secretary and your boss will scold you.

## Admitting, Discharging and Transferring Patients

All these may seem daunting when you first qualify, but the task can be made very simple by having a small checklist for each one. You need to provide enough information so that any doctor 'off the street' (for example a locum who has never seen the patient before) could meet the patient, read the notes and then treat the patient for their condition. The reason for this is simple – safety. You may not always be around when the condition of the patient deteriorates suddenly and if you have not documented what you have diagnosed and what treatment plan you have instigated then the patient's care or, more severely, life may be put at risk. This applies equally well to patients being admitted from the A&E department as it does to patients being discharged from the day surgery unit. If all the criteria are fulfilled then it is safe to change the location of the patient (Tables 4.3 and 4.4).

**Table 4.3** Admission checklist

| Checklist | Description |
| --- | --- |
| History and examination | Written account of your clerking. |
| Investigations requested and any results | List the investigations requested and any results available. This particularly applies to blood results. If you know them, then write them in the notes so it is clear. It is good practice to do this, as when you are tired it is easy to misread values from the computer. Writing them down means they have to be processed through your brain first. Every doctor has made this mistake at least once, usually by reading the wrong line for haemoglobin or electrolytes which can result in serious consequences the next day. The key phrase is 'if it is worth requesting an investigation, it is worth waiting for and documenting the result'. |
| Diagnosis and treatment plan | You may obviously need to discuss this with your seniors. |
| Drug chart | Prescribe all the patients regular medications plus analgesia and intravenous fluids if necessary. This will prevent you being disturbed in the night for the sake of the patient wishing to have two paracetamol tablets. If you are prescribing opioids then add laxatives too. |
| Bed manager | Inform them of your intention to admit the patient. This can be done directly or, if admitting from the A&E department it is sometimes performed by the nursing staff. You will need to let them know which is the preferred ward to admit them to. |
| Ward nurses | Let them know about the expected ward admission so they can prepare. They will need to know the diagnosis and your treatment plan, plus any special care that will need to be administered over the next few hours. |
| Admission list | Once all the above is done, keep a note of the patient's details, diagnosis, ward and any results that need checking. Your SpR will want to look at this list during your on-call and it will be required on the post take ward round. |

**Table 4.4** Discharge checklist

| Checklist | Description |
|---|---|
| TTAs | As outlined in the take away sheets section. |
| Follow-up appointment | The patient may need to be seen in the out-patients clinic, at a review clinic in the A&E department or fracture clinic. |
| Discharge summary | This is usually written by the SpR or SHO on the firm, but there should be a brief summary on the TTAs. |
| Further out-patient investigations | Some patients may require additional investigation before attending for follow-up or a simple blood examination in the few days after discharge. Hospital investigations should be requested and booked with a date (some departments send the appointment for the investigation through the post after the request has been made). Arrange other simple tests by telephoning the GP and politely asking him or her to organise them for you. If you are unable to speak to the GP then leave a message for the GP to call you. Do not assume the GP has received the message. Instead always ask for confirmation. In both cases the patient should always be aware of which investigations are necessary and the dates of when they are to be performed (they are more likely to remember that something has not been done than you or their GP). In the case of blood tests, ask the patient to attend the GP on a particular day after arranging this with the GP. |
| Wound care | If a patient has a wound, either surgical or an ulcer, then this may need care after discharge, that is removal of sutures and dressings. Commonly this will be the done via the district nurse if the patient is poorly mobile or by the GP nurse if mobile. The ward nurses will arrange this after you have discussed your requirements with them. |

The transferring procedure can vary from place to place, but generally if you are transferring the patient to another ward under the care of another consultant then a simple written summary in the notes of the patient's admission will suffice. However, if the patient is being transferred to another hospital it is customary to provide the features shown in Table 4.5.

## Ward Layout/Putting Things Back

Each hospital has a different ward layout, but generally all wards are the same within a hospital in architectural terms. However, where individual items are stored varies widely and depends on the ward sister who ultimately decides where things go. It is extremely important to be aware where everyday equipment, notes and emergency

Table 4.5 Transfer checklist

| Checklist | Description |
|---|---|
| TTAs | These may be required, particularly if a patient is going to another hospital or to a rehabilitation unit. |
| Follow-up appointment | The patient may need to be seen in the out-patients clinic unless they are going to be followed up at the receiving hospital. |
| Transfer letter | A basic typed summary of the patient's admission outlining the reason for admission, treatment given and course of recovery. This is very similar to a discharge summary but often written by the PRHO or SHO instead. |
| Results of recent investigations | Your letter should list recent blood results and any other relevant investigation results. |
| Photocopies of the hospital notes | These are sometimes required and you should always ask your seniors before sending this type of confidential information out of the hospital. It is potentially a breach of doctor–patient confidentiality. You should never send originals, as these are the property of the hospital trust. |

equipment are kept on each ward where you work. This is obvious stuff. Most juniors need to know the basics such as where the patient notes and radiographs are kept and where request forms and the phlebotomy equipment is. Occasionally you will require equipment for performing a neurological or ENT examination. In theory there should be a tray on all wards containing all the necessary items, kept by the nursing staff. More often than not items are stolen, lost or broken and it is necessary to borrow these missing items from the relevant specialist ward. When doing so, you will require identification and must return the items when you have finished. I have spent many frustrating hours hunting round wards for something as simple as a tendon hammer in the middle of the night and ended up using the end of my stethoscope instead. Hardly satisfactory when you think your patient may have had a stroke and you need to refer them to the on-call medical SpR.

## Consent

Consent, from the Latin *consentire* meaning 'agree', is defined as to 'give permission' or 'agree to do'.[1] However, 'informed consent' is what we really mean with regards to

---

[1] *Oxford English Dictionary*. Oxford: Oxford University Press; 1973.

the medical profession. To ask informed consent, you, the person obtaining the consent, must be

- skilled in performing the procedure for which you are obtaining consent
- aware of the reasons for undertaking the procedure
- aware of the possible alternatives
- aware of the complications
- aware of the risks versus benefits, that is the risk of action
- aware of the risk of not having the procedure, that is the risk of inaction

For this reason, only SHOs who are experienced or more senior staff should obtain consent for the majority of procedures and all operations.

Obtaining informed consent for surgery is beyond the experience and skill of the PRHO and is therefore illegal.[2] You should not be asked to do so and, if you are, you should politely refuse explaining why. If you are obtaining informed consent for any other procedure (for example a chest drain insertion) you should fulfil the criteria listed above. If you feel unable to obtain consent then you should not be performing the procedure unsupervised.

When performing any procedure to which you have obtained verbal informed consent, which is most often the case (for example a central line insertion, chest drain insertion, pleural tap, etc.), this should be written in the patients medical notes as follows: 'Verbal informed consent obtained. Risks explained (list them).'

## Performing Procedures

It is not uncommon for an enthusiastic PRHO to perform a multitude of practical procedures during their two posts, particularly in district general hospitals. This will be at the request of your seniors or you may have decided that it is clinically appropriate yourself. If this is the case, however, it should always be discussed with your senior, unless it is very clear-cut (for example urinary catheterisation for acute retention of urine).

Examples of the procedures a PRHO may be expected to perform after proper instruction and understanding of the task (the 'see one, do one, teach one' rule is applied with alarming regularity) are listed below.

- urinary catheterisation
- arterial blood sampling
- nasogastric tube insertion
- chest drain insertion

---

[2] General Medical Council.

- pleural fluid aspiration/tap
- abdominal paracentesis
- central/femoral/long peripheral line insertion
- lumbar puncture
- simple suturing of wounds
- removal of a surgical drain

As explained already, the first step is obtaining informed consent. Once the patient has agreed to the procedure you need to set up the appropriate equipment on a stainless steel trolley. Often for certain procedures a kind member of nursing staff will set up the trolley for you, but do not expect this as it is not the 'norm'. If the trolley has been set up for you it is vitally important to check you have everything you need before you begin. It is common for small but important items to be missed. Once you are alone with the patient and have donned a pair of sterile gloves and set your kit up, you will look and feel highly unprofessional if you are missing something. Not only will you lose 'face', but you can put the patient at risk.

> *The commonest omission I have come across is not having a 10-ml ampoule of sterile saline/water to fill up the catheter balloon or having no syringe with which to inject it. As an inexperienced PRHO in the middle of the night catheterising a man in acute retention of urine I have on several occasions forgotten to fill the syringe in advance, as the patient being in agony has distracted me. In my rush to catheterise them I have found myself in the compromising position of having urine flowing freely into the bag (if you have remembered to connect it beforehand else it flows onto the bed and then the floor), but have nothing to fill the balloon. One must then either get the patient to hold their own catheter in while you run off to get some saline or a syringe (they are usually so distracted they are incapable of this) or call a nurse from the next bay who will usually not hear. Shouting across the ward from behind curtains in the middle of the night often (1) makes you feel stupid, (2) embarrasses the patient, (3) alarms the nursing staff and (4) wakes up the other patients.*

Always check once, then check twice and, if you are tired or inexperienced, run through the procedure in you head and check again.

During the procedure maintain sterility at all times and, if inexperienced, always ask a senior or a PRHO who is more experienced than you to either supervise or assist you. Do not feel embarrassed if you have to ask your SHO or SpR to supervise you several times, even if they become annoyed.

The basic rule is, if you are not confident, do not perform the procedure, as your mistake may have more serious consequences than the initial reason for performing it. It is better to irritate your senior by getting them out of bed to perform a procedure that you are not confident with than cause iatrogenic pathology.

*I have seen PRHOs and SHOs who are not fully happy with their skills or overconfident performing pleural taps or chest drain insertions for pleural effusions. This has on more than several occasions resulted in the patient sustaining iatrogenic haemothorax, pneumothorax or both. This can lead to a life-threatening situation so beware. I have attended a cardiac arrest call for a life-threatening iatrogenic haemothorax secondary to a pleural tap (which thankfully I did not perform, but it can so easily happen to any of us). There was one stupidly simple reason it was not diagnosed earlier – the PRHO who had performed the tap had not written that the tap was 'bloodstained' in the notes. The lesson here is that good documentation saves lives. Had the documentation been better the diagnosis would have been made earlier and the patient would have been treated before becoming critically unwell.*

When performing the procedure keep a mental note of the quantity and type of sharps used. After you have finished clear away your mess – it is your responsibility. Again, a kind nurse may offer to do it for you, in which case accept gladly and then go to write in the notes. However, you should bear in mind that it is your legal responsibility to clear away your own sharps into the sharps box. When disposing of them make sure your mental tally is in keeping with the number you dispose of. If a nurse clears up for you, inform them of the number of sharps on the trolley. This is good practice and the nurse will thank you for it.

Lastly, you need to make a note of the procedure in the patient's notes. You should title the procedure and underline it. The date, time and your name, grade and bleep number are all requirements. Mention the degree of sterility and anatomical approach (see Figure 4.1).

> It is important as a PRHO and SHO to try and follow up any patient on whom you have performed a procedure in order to see what the outcome was. If they had a complication was it something that you did badly or was the patient simply very unwell? Could you have done anything differently to change their outcome? This is the first step to auditing your own 'outcome measures' and a very good learning exercise. For example, if you are not sure whether your 'sterile technique' was sterile enough, did the patient get an infection afterwards?

## How to Deal with the Death of Your Patient

Death is more common than you may expect (particularly in some specialities such as elderly medicine or vascular surgery) and it is always emotionally difficult. Some of you may have experienced it as a medical student when a patient you have clerked

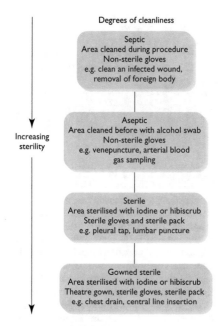

Degrees of cleanliness

Septic
Area cleaned during procedure
Non-sterile gloves
e.g. clean an infected wound,
removal of foreign body

Aseptic
Area cleaned before with alcohol swab
Non-sterile gloves
e.g. venepuncture, arterial blood
gas sampling

Increasing
sterility

Sterile
Area sterilised with iodine or hibiscrub
Sterile gloves and sterile pack
e.g. pleural tap, lumbar puncture

Gowned sterile
Area sterilised with iodine or hibiscrub
Theatre gown, sterile gloves, sterile pack
e.g. chest drain, central line insertion

**Figure 4.1** Types of procedure cleanliness.

died. The feeling of loss and lack of power is the same when you are qualified, only magnified. This is because you spend a lot more time with your patients than when an undergraduate and, more importantly, you see their relatives and treat the patient for their disease. Often for the first time you realise that your patients fit into a family network as you do and that, when they die, it affects everyone. It is difficult when you have been trying to treat disease but the patient is overwhelmed and deteriorates. The important thing is to do what you can.

It is natural to be upset, but you must remember that the only certain thing in life is death. Whether a person dies or not is not always the most important thing – this may sound strange. More importantly is how the patient dies – are they with family, are they comfortable and dignified, or are they alone and suffering in pain and distress fighting for breath?

Dignity and lack of suffering above all else is paramount. Patients should absolutely not die in pain or distress although on rare occasions this does happen. You should take it upon yourself to make sure patients receive analgesia and anxiolysis where necessary to release them from pain and suffering (and by release I do not mean euthanasia). Relatives should be fully aware of the events leading up to death and you will find that, if you have explained things well to their relatives, it will be easier for you and them to deal with it. There is no feeling on Earth worse than knowing you let someone die without doing all you could for your patient or their relatives.

## Death Certificates

All medical students now have to be formally taught how to fill in these forms. The basic details are not difficult, but most newly qualified doctors get stuck on the cause of death (Ia, Ib, Ic and II). The most important thing to remember is to ask your seniors if you are unsure, but as a PRHO you should not be filling in the cause of death without discussing it with your seniors. You should remember that 'arrest' or 'failure' of a physiological system is not a legitimate cause of death, for example cardiac arrest, cardiac failure and renal failure. You must state the cause of the failure. If there is any doubt the cause of death should be discussed with the coroner (see below).

It is important that you write your name and bleep number in capital letters on the certificate and the stub by your signature (Figure 4.2). This enables you to be traced by hospital staff, relatives or the coroner if there are any queries regarding the cause of death. It is good medical practice to identify yourself every time you write on patient notes (see the section on clinical governance).

## Cremation Forms

This is a legal form in which you give your medical opinion that the body is not required for any further medical investigation (that is autopsy) and that there is no doubt as to the cause of death (Figure 4.3). Furthermore, you must state that the body contains no substances that may be harmful when burnt (for example a pacemaker, which explodes quite dramatically, radioactive substances, which disperse or inflatable orthopaedic nails, which are not dangerous but explode with a very loud bang). Once you have filled the form identifying yourself clearly, the form is sent to patient affairs where the relatives pick up a copy of the form and give it to the funeral directors. The undertaker must present this form to the mortuary officer in order to collect the body for cremation. No body may be cremated in the UK without a properly filled cremation form. Once the undertaker has collected the body he will leave a cheque for you with patient affairs to cover the cost of your time. This is colloquially known as 'ash cash'. The amount varies from region to region, but is usually approximately £45–55. In some trusts a percentage is skimmed off, which goes directly into the mess fund or, on rare occasions, all ash cash goes directly to the mess fund (hard luck – I hope you get some good parties!).

## The Coroner and Post-mortems

Many juniors perceive the coroner as a scary person who will berate you when you telephone him or her because you have let your patient die. In actual fact the coroner is simply another doctor who works to establish the cause of death in patients where there is doubt or if the patient has had an accident, operation or violent insult prior to death. Most often coroners are very friendly and obliging people who are more than happy to talk to you and discuss the death of your patient. Usually when you get through you will talk to the coroner's assistant who will require certain details before handing you on to the coroner. Increasingly, it is the coroner's assistant who decides whether or not you actually need to speak to the coroner and these assistants can occasionally be a little supercilious. When you telephone, have the following details to hand.

- name and address of the patient
- date of birth and the time and date of death
- date of and reason for admission to hospital
- mode of admission, for example GP referral, via the A&E department or elective admission
- in-patient diagnoses and treatment
- background medical history
- what you think the cause of death was that you are intending to write on the death certificate, that is Ia, Ib, Ic and II
- name and telephone number of the next of kin

There are certain times when it is mandatory to report the death of a patient to the coroner, for example death due to an accident or violence. These are changing with time and the patient affairs or bereavement affairs office in your hospital can provide you with an up-to-date list.

## Dress Code and Personal Hygiene

### Clothes
All professionals should dress appropriately, particularly doctors. Men should wear clean, ironed shirts and trousers (not combats) and a tie. Men should shave daily

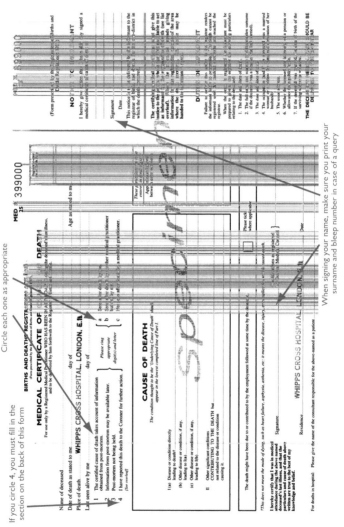

Figure 4.2a Death certificate, side A. Sections are self-explanatory, but some require explanation as shown.

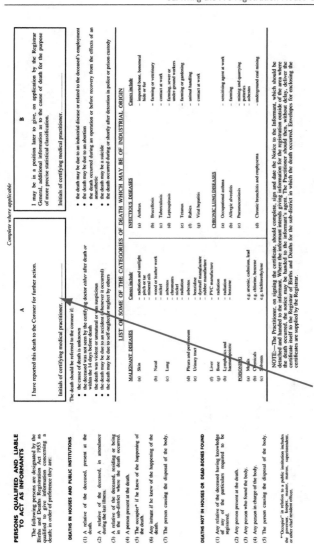

Sign here if you have discussed the death with the coroner. Note that if a post mortem is required, you will not be filling out the death certificate as the cause of death is not yet established.

Figure 4.2b Death certificate, side B.

This form is issued by the
London Borough of Haringey,
Cemeteries & Crematorium Dept.
Enfield Crematorium,
Gt. Cambridge Road, Enfield
0181-363 8324/5

**Form
B, C & F**

**CREMATION ACT, 1902**
*Statutory Rules and Orders, 1930*

These Forms are Statutory, All the questions must be answered, therefore, to make the Certificate effective for the purposes of Cremation.

These medical certificates are regarded as strictly confidential. The right to inspect them is confined to the Secretary of State, the Ministry of Health, and the Chief Officer of a Police Force.

**Form B.**

**CERTIFICATE OF MEDICAL ATTENDANT**

(1) This form is not to be used in the case of a Coroner's Inquest.

I am informed that application is about to be made for the cremation of the remains of:-

(Name of Deceased).............................

(Address).............................

(2) Note:- The answers to the question should be as concise as possible. Figures may be used instead of words. All the questions must be answered.

(Occupation or Description).............................(Age)............

Having attended the Deceased before death, and seen and identified the body after death I give the following answers to the questions set out below:-

1. On what date, and at what hour, did he or she die?

2. What was the place where the deceased died?
   (Give address and say whether own residence, lodging, hotel, hospital, nursing home, etc.).

   *Give the ward and hospital*

3. Are you a relative of the deceased? If so, state the relationship.

4. Have you, so far as you are aware, any pecuniary interest in the death of the deceased?

   *This means you will gain financially from the death of the patient. The answer should be "No"*

5. (a) Were you the ordinary medical attendant of the deceased?

   (a)...... *The ordinary medical attendant is the GP*

   (b) If so, for how long?

   (b)...... *As the hospital doctor, you should write "No"*

6. (a) Did you attend the deceased during his or her last illness?

   (a).............................

   (b) If so, for how long?

   (b).............................

7. When did you last see the deceased alive?
   (Say how many days or hours before death)

8. (a) How soon after death did you see the body?

   (The doctor must see the body after death)

   (a).............................

   (b) What examination did it did you make?

   (b)...... *Your examination should be external only*

8A. If the deceased died in a hospital* at which he or she was an in-patient, has a post-mortem examination been made by a registered medical practitioner of not less than five years' standing who is neither a relative of the deceased not a relative or partner of yours and are the results of that examination known to you?

   *Has a post mortem been performed?
   Answer "Yes" or "No"*

(3) If the death has been reported to Coroner for any reason, this should be stated in answer to question 18.

9. What was the cause of death?
   (I)
   Immediate cause

   (a).............................

   Morbid conditions, if any, giving rise to immediate cause (stated in order proceeding backwards from immediate cause).

   due to
   (b)...... *This should read the same
   as the Death Certificate*

   due to
   (c).............................

   (II)
   Other morbid conditions (if important) contributing to death but not related to immediate cause.

   .............................
   .............................

   *(over)*

Figure 4.3a A cremation form.

| | | |
|---|---|---|
| 10. | (a) What was the mode of death? Say whether syncope, coma, exhaustion, convulsions, etc) | (a) <u>e.g. cardiac arrest, respiratory arrest</u> |
| | (b) What was its duration in days, hours, or minutes? | (b)........................................................... |
| 11. | State how far the answers to the last *two* questions are the result of your own observations, or are based on statements made by others. If on statements made by others, say by whom. | If you have been looking after the patient it is usually sufficient to say "own" but you can add "nursing staff on ward" as well |
| 12. | (a) Did the deceased undergo any operation during the final illness or within a year before death? | (a)....................................... "Yes" or "No" |
| | (b) If so, what was its nature and who performed it? | List the operation and surgeon (e.g. nephrectomy (b)............................ for renal carcinoma. Mr L. Ureter) |
| 13. | By whom was the deceased nursed during his or her last illness? (Give names, and say whether professional nurse, relative etc. If the illness was a long one, this question should be answered with reference to the period of four weeks before the death). | Nursing staff on ward |
| 14. | Who were the persons (if any ) present at the moment of death? | Relatives or nurses. It is inadvisable to state that the patient died alone |
| 15. | In view of the knowledge of the deceased's habits and constitution, do you feel any doubts whatever as to the character of the deceased or the cause of death? | "No" |
| 16. | Have you any reason to suspect that the death of the deceased was due, directly or indirectly, to (a) Violence..................... "No" (b) Poison........................ "No" (c) Privation or neglect?.... "No" | *Death due directly to alcohol has now to be reported to the Coroner* |
| 17. | Have you any reason whatever to suppose a further examination of the body to be desirable? | "No" |
| (4) When the certificate for registration has been given by authority of the Coroner, this fact should be stated. | 18. Have you given the certificate required for registration of death? If not, who has? | |

**I Hereby Certify** that the answers given above are true and accurate to the best of my knowledge and belief, and that I know of no reasonable cause to suspect that the deceased died either a violent or an unnatural death or a sudden death of which the cause is unknown or died in such place or circumstances as to require an inquest in pursuance of any act.

Name in BLOCK
LETTERS please ......................................................... *(Signature)* ...........................................................

**IMPORTANT**
Addendum — Form "B"
(a) Has the deceased been fitted with a cardiac pacemaker or radioactive implant? YES/NO
(b) If answer to (a) is in the affirmative has this been removed? YES/NO

*(Address)*...........................................................

*(Registered Qualifications)*....e.g. BSc, MBBS

*(Date)*................................ *(Tel.)*...........................

Please delete as applicable.

NOTE:- *This certificate must be handed or sent in a closed envelope by the medical practitioner who signs it to the medical practitioner who is to give the confirmatory certificate below.*

*The bearer of the certificate can act as the agent of the medical attendant, and to him may be handed the closed envelope for delivery to the other medical practitioner, except in a case where question 8A above is answered in the affirmative, in which case the certificate must be so handed or sent to the Medical Referee.*

*\*The term "Hospital" as used here means any institution for the reception and treatment of persons suffering from illness or mental disorder, any maternity home, and any institution for the reception and treatment of persons during convalescence.*

It is mandatory to circle YES or NO on (a) and (b) to allow cremation.
NB: radioactive implants, pacemakers and inflatable orthopaedic nails explode and are potentially harmful and must be removed prior to cremation by the undertakers or morticians

**Figure 4.3b**

unless post on-call. It is not acceptable to turn up to ward rounds or meetings with relatives looking like you have not left the hospital for three days. (It may be that you have not actually left the hospital for three days but you should try not to look like it if possible!) I have seen patients hold their breath while being examined on the post take ward round because doctors have not washed or changed their clothes since the previous day. If you are prone to body odour and your shirt smells, then bring a spare when on-call or wear theatre blues and change them in the morning. Women should wear trousers or skirt with an appropriate top (not exposing too much cleavage) as it draws the attention of not only your male colleagues but also the patients!

### Footwear

Only two rules apply – no trainers and no open-toed shoes. However, both of these are flouted relentlessly! The reasons for the rule are simple – health and safety. Trainers are porous and allow body fluids to penetrate. Open-toed shoes are a sharps disaster waiting to happen. Although open-toed shoes, sandals, etc. are banned in most hospitals, most female doctors can get away with wearing anything they wish (you know it is true). The decision is very much up to the individual. I have seen two female PRHOs get needle stick injuries in their feet that were preventable. The first was by dropping a needle and syringe and the second was by stubbing a toe on a needle at a medical emergency.

Most juniors (myself included) often wear trainers with surgical scrubs when on surgical take (particularly nights) as they are more comfortable and easier to run in (to trauma calls/emergencies), but as you become more senior you spend less time on the ward at night and so have less need for them. However, when you are standing up for most of the day and night spending long hours in uncomfortable theatre clogs, most people find trainers a real pleasure! Just do not turn up to the post take ward round in them or you will probably feel your consultant's shoe leather on a certain posterior aspect of your anatomy. This is usually a very effective method of your boss conveying which type of shoes he or she prefers you to wear.

# 5

# The Team

## The Department

As explained before, each trust is divided up into clinical departments led by a clinical director, for example a directorate of surgery or university department of surgery in a teaching hospital. The head of department is usually the most senior doctor or in a teaching hospital a professor. Each department is further divided into clinical and non-clinical staff who must all interact at a professional and personal level to ensure the smooth and efficient running of the department (Figure 5.1).

## The Firm

The word 'firm' has been used in this text already. Within each medical and surgical department there are several teams or 'firms', which are usually led by a single consultant with a specialist field. These firms are simply a group of doctors who provide care for their group of patients. Occasionally two consultants may join forces to produce a single large firm, for example respiratory, urology or vascular surgery. Each firm has its own specialist registrar (SpR), senior house officer (SHO) and/or pre-registration house officer (PRHO). In the case of a double firm there may be an SpR for each consultant and the SHO and PRHO work for both.

A firm usually runs from a group of specialist wards, but nursing staff work for the ward and not the firm. The purpose of having specialist wards is to concentrate expertise in one field to one place in the hospital and therefore increase the excellence of care, as patients have faster access to specialist doctors, nurses and professionals allied to medicine (now called allied health professionals: see the chapter on therapists and professionals allied to medicine) and it has been shown that there are fewer clinical errors in these settings.

As a PRHO you are expected to run your firm. This means that you are responsible for the organisation and day-to-day running of things. You must generate and maintain an up-to-date patient list and generate and submit theatre lists as well as request, organise and get the results of in- and out-patient investigations.

Nursing staff work for a ward and therefore care for patients under any firm regardless of speciality. However, as most wards have a particular speciality the bed and ward managers try to keep patients on the ward restricted to certain consultants. In times of bed crises it is not unusual to find your patients all over the hospital. This is often a source of much time wasting and frustration trying to hunt down patients admitted from the previous day's take. If you have come in early and know where all the patients are, your consultant will be impressed by your diligence.

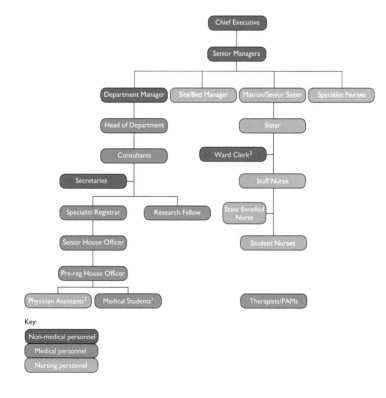

**Figure 5.1** The medical team.

[1] Medical students: note that they are as much a part of the team and department as qualified doctors and should have specific roles set out in the firm. They can be a source of much fun, entertainment and flirtation. Medical students, depending on their year of study, are a valuable resource. Most can perform venepuncture, cannulation, clerk and, to a point, diagnose. Not only can they be clinically useful, but they can help with organising meetings and often will learn more about the patients than junior doctors will as they have more time. As doctors will remember from being a student, patients often open up to and tell students their worries, as they do not wish 'to bother the doctor'. They can therefore provide useful clinical input into the management of the patients.

[2] Physician assistants: nowadays, most firms have an assistant whose role varies from firm to firm. All assistants are capable of taking blood and chasing scans/radiographs, etc. and should be used as much as possible to save on your time, allowing you to devote it to your patients. Often they have cannulation skills too. At the beginning of your post it is a good idea to sit down with your assistant (if you have one) and discuss their role. Should there be anything you think they could be doing that they do not already do then discuss it with them. More often than not they are willing to expand their role to give them more responsibility. Once you have established a good relationship, you will find it very valuable.

[3] Ward clerk: this person is usually very helpful and friendly, being more than willing to help newly qualified stressed out doctors. Their job is to run the administrative side of the ward, ordering notes from medical records for elective patients, organising medical notes and filing investigation results, etc. Depending on which hospital you work in, some ward clerks organise writing the basics on the to take away sheets (patient name, GP and admission dates), which will save you time. If you are borrowing notes and radiographs from the ward for meetings or referrals then the ward clerk is the person you should inform first so they can be booked out. Keep on the friendly side of these people, as you will regret making them angry – they can make your life on the ward hell if you are arrogant and obnoxious to them.

**KEY:** Dark blue – non-medical personnel; mid blue – medical personnel; pale blue – nursing personnel.

# 6

# Your Consultant: Keeping Them Happy

## Roles and Responsibilities of the Boss

This may seem very obvious and you are probably asking yourself why have I written this section. The answer is quite simple: consultants are rapidly losing their autonomy and with the new consultant contract things are set to get worse. In the 'good old days' consultants could generally dedicate their life to a field of their interest, combining both National Health Service and private work. Research was performed by the interested and most good senior doctors audited their own patient treatment outcomes. Litigation was low and politicians were kept at arms length.

In recent years the amount of time spent doing useful clinical work has decreased and the amount of time spent doing managerial or political type work has increased. This is to the dissatisfaction of most consultants who enjoy being doctors rather than managers. The role of the consultant is slowly changing and this is what concerns and frustrates most of them. Consultants are now in constant liaison with hospital managers and the chief executive over department funding and government targets with regard to clinical incidents, complaints and litigation, research and audit and waiting times for clinics or operations.

When you see your consultant is not happy you should ask yourself why: have they just opened their mail to discover they have to attain a new and medically useless target or have they had another argument with the chief executive over funding?

## Staffing: Permanent Staff Versus Fluid Staff

Staffing is a major issue and worry for any consultant. It is difficult for juniors to imagine the constant flux of staff through a department and the effect it has on both patient care and staff morale. Junior medical staff (that is pre-registration house officers

(PRHOs) and senior house officers (SHOs)) rotate every six months and senior medical staff (special registrars (SpRs)) every 12–18 months, occasionally longer. Each rotating junior needs to be taught how the hospital and firm runs at the beginning of each six months and only become fully competent towards the end of their post. This is demoralising for nursing staff to know that the good doctors leave, only to be replaced by another with less skill and knowledge (in that particular field!). Juniors should note that nursing staff often move and rotate too, particularly in London.

> You will notice when you start work that your consultant may be far more at ease with senior nurses and doctors than with you. This is not a personal issue, but simply that senior medical and nursing staff are more static and therefore have known each other longer. You will also find that they constitute the backbone of the department. Therefore, you should pay attention to and respect them.

## What Does Your Consultant Need from Their Pre-Registration House Officer?

More than anything else, a junior needs to be easy to get on with and should be reliable. It is often thought that the most intelligent person is the best junior. This is a common misperception. It is far more important to be an adaptable and agreeable person than a 'grade A' student, as most consultants will teach you what they want you to know and the way they want things done. They want you to be able to be polite and courteous to their patients and get on with the nursing staff. Timekeeping and efficiency are just as important.

Also known affectionately as the 'houseplant', the houseman is the ward all rounder who is expected to do anything and manage the more 'basic' tasks on the ward. I use the word basic very loosely as often the PRHO is the most important member of the team who will deal with more urgent and life-threatening problems more often than, and before anyone else on the team. The PRHO should be able to manage most ward-based tasks and liaise with seniors when out of their depth.

> Probably the single most important skill a junior should acquire from day 1 is the ability to know when they are out of their depth and not be afraid or embarrassed to call a more senior colleague. This skill, if learnt early, will save lives.

The PRHO should be able to keep patients and their relatives informed of all treatment plans and upcoming investigations as well as results. You should run the ward round (a very important part of the running of the firm) and be able to lead your consultant around each patient and be able to relate the clinical history for each one. The easiest way to do this is to make a list of patients with the latest blood and other investigation results. If you are able to present a clear clinical picture for each patient your consultant will be smiling by the end of the round and will invariably buy the whole team coffee (and if you are lucky a cake/doughnut!). If not, then you are likely to be shouted at and go thirsty as well as embarrassed (yes, I do speak from experience!).

## Why Your Consultant Does Not Know Your Name

Juniors can often find that the boss is distracted and stressed a lot of the time, or that he or she does not engage in day-to-day conversation with juniors. This is often difficult for juniors to accept, as the consultant is usually jovial and friendly with the SpR. This is because juniors rotate every six months and the consultant has little time to get to know you. Just take five minutes to work out how many weeks you will actually work for the boss in your six-month job (based on a partial or full shift rota) ... any guesses? ... then read on.

Add up one half day a week (which most of us do not actually manage to get), a week of nights followed by a week off every six to eight weeks. Three weeks of annual leave, a week of sick leave (approximately) and one week of study leave. In the end you will only spend 11–12 weeks out of 24 weeks with your consultant. Bear in mind that this means you only get 11–12 weeks of training from your team!

With increasing age, most consultants give up trying to get to know their juniors for this very reason and appear less friendly. However, it is simply that they do not have the time or energy and their mind is concentrating on other matters. As consultants become more senior their political and economic targets increase. SpRs, on the other hand, stay for 12 months or more and spend more time with the consultant in theatre and clinics, etc.

## What You Can Do to Ease the Pressure

There are certain things that the junior can do to break down barriers that are very effective. Most surgeons listen to music in theatre when operating and offering to bring in a CD can prove very effective at generating conversation. Engage in conversation at appropriate times with any consultant, for example during ward rounds or clinics (as long as you are not in earshot of any patients or their relatives). Most importantly, let your consultant get to know and trust you. Once there is trust between you, you will be allowed to practise more freely and be taught a lot more.

# 7

# Nurses

Nurses can be a tricky bunch, having spent years on the wards gaining experience only to be belittled by arrogant newly qualified doctors. You will see colleagues trying this approach and notice that it does not work, and furthermore, that they will quickly gain a reputation around the hospital. No-one will explain when you are in medical school that qualified nurses are a valuable asset. They can be your best ally or worst enemy depending on how you treat them. Most often they have been working in a particular speciality (for example orthopaedics, urology, etc.) for many years and, while set in their ways, have a vast knowledge of the usual treatment practices that you will need for managing your patients successfully. Coming straight out of medical school or house jobs you may have more theoretical knowledge of physiology, pharmacology, etc., but your ward experience will be limited. Nursing staff will be able to guide you through the prescriber's minefield reminding you of times and doses when you are trying to write up drugs on a ward round (a word of caution: always check the *British National Formulary* if in any doubt whatsoever). The nurses will also know the way each particular consultant likes his/her patients managed.

Nurses can be your best friend and your worst enemy, often within minutes of each other if you say the wrong thing at the wrong time. Historically, doctors have always thought themselves more hard done-by than any other medical professionals and as a response to this have always seen themselves as superior to nursing staff, both in their educational/intellectual level or in status. Nowadays more than ever before, nurses and doctors need to work side by side as equals in the workplace although ultimately the overall responsibility and duty of care of the patient rests with the doctor. This responsibility can often cause problems, as some junior nursing (and occasionally older) staff do not realise this concept. When giving instructions regarding the care of patients there is often debate between doctors and nursing staff, which can look unprofessional and not be in the best interests of the patient. See the section on giving instructions on how to handle this.

Nurses are not there to help you. They have their own role, just as you are not on the ward for their benefit. Nurses and doctors work together as a team for a common goal: the care and treatment of the patients. There are grey areas between the responsibilities of nursing and doctoring (for example setting up catheter/central line trolleys, etc.). Nursing staff will often do these things for you if you are busy and they are not, if you ask them nicely. However, always double-check the trolley first, as they sometimes forget small but important items.

For those of you interested in sport I have an analogy for you. Pony trekking or horse riding can be dangerous, as can caring for patients. Horses, like nurses, are intelligent and can be trained. They also have the ability to think, assess situations and come to a decision. When a new rider gets on a horse, the horse will test the rider to see how experienced they are or how in control the rider is by trying to eat grass or wander off the track, going too slowly, etc. The horse needs to have confidence in their rider and once this relationship is established the horse and rider make a good team. The ride is more accurate and faster with less hesitancy. Overall you are less likely to fall off and therefore the whole ride is safer.

You can see the parallel with nurses: they need to be confident in your actions and judgement before they will let you do things alone without question. You need to have mutual respect and trust in each other to know that, when the nurse bleeps you, that it is for something important. Likewise when you ask a nurse to do something it is equally important that you can trust that they will do it. Once this relationship is established the ward runs more smoothly, quickly and efficiently. The time you spend on the ward will be better spent and therefore you will get more time to sip coffee in the mess. When you have this relationship with nursing staff, the patient care will improve and less clinical errors will occur.

I thought this was the perfect analogy but, in retrospect, I think it is flawed in one area. In this analogy, the rider is the master and the horse does what it is told. This is absolutely not true of the relationship between doctors and nurses. Nurses are a profession in their own right and, therefore, I think I should give you another example.

In rowing the oarsmen can propel the boat in relative safety without the need for a coxswain. However, with a coxswain to give some direction the winning combination is made. The coxswain has the overall responsibility of the boat and is able to see what is up ahead and can assess the situation and alter the direction of the boat. However, without the oarsmen the coxswain would go nowhere. Medicine is a little like this: the doctor is responsible for the overall care of the patient but the nursing staff do the majority of the work. The nursing staff are capable of caring for the patient without a doctor, but together the patient is more likely to recover.

## Ten Things Doctors Do That Nurses Hate

1 Leave sharps lying around – this is a sackable offence. It is your responsibility to dispose of your own sharps. Likewise, do not clear up someone else's sharps, as if you are unlucky enough to sustain a sharps injury you may not be able to trace the donor.

2 Leave writing to take away (TTA) sheets until a few hours before the patient is due for discharge.

3 Leave rewriting drug charts until they are full so nurses cannot dispense the patients' medications.

4 Mis-communicating or not communicating information to nurses, patients and their relatives. The most effective way to decrease National Health Service (NHS) expenditure is to improve communication. This in turn decreases clinical error and thus, litigation (see the section on giving instructions).

5 Not certifying patients deceased rapidly so they can be sent to the mortuary.

6 Borrowing notes or radiographs without letting the senior nursing or ward administrative staff know.

7 Being arrogant or not admitting you are in the wrong.

8 Thinking you know more than you do (see point 7). This is extremely dangerous and one of the most common causes of clinical mistakes. If in doubt ask a senior.

9 Not answering your bleep within a reasonable time. Most nurses expect junior doctors to answer within approximately five to ten seconds (as we have nothing better to do and will obviously be sitting by the telephone in the doctor's mess). However unrealistic their expectations, you should not take longer than one minute to answer your bleep unless you are performing a procedure or talking to relatives, etc. In this situation, try and ask someone to hold your bleep until you are finished.

10 Expect a nurse to set up a trolley for you so you can perform a practical proced-ure (see the section on performing procedures).

11 Last one, promise! Not visiting the ward before you go to bed when on-call. If there is a good night sister on (and they usually are) then they will amass a num-ber of non-urgent jobs that need doing before you turn in, for example cannula-tion, reading electrocardiographs and checking observation readings. They will often not bleep you for these as they are not 'urgent', but require doing before bed. It is good practice to drop in to each of your wards before bed to (i) clear up any jobs and (ii) let the nurses know so they do not bleep you too much. Most nurses appreciate that doctors need their sleep too and will try to minimise the number of bleeps they make if they know you have gone to bed.

## Ten Things Nurses Do That Doctors Hate

1 Bleeping you more than once for the same minor task.

2 Bleeping you 'just to let you know …': you can avoid the majority of these calls by setting a threshold limit for the nurses to call you, for example bleep me if Mr Smith's systolic drops below 100 mmHg, oxygen saturations drop below 94%, etc.

3 Bleep you and then immediately walk away from the telephone.

4 Not take a verbal prescription order for intravenous fluids or simple analgesia over the telephone.

5 Not set up a trolley with all the kit you need after they have offered to do it for you or set it up but do not give you everything you need.

6 Ask you to do jobs just before you are supposed to go home or when you are not on-call. In these cases, diplomacy and patience are the only way forward. You will often want to wring someone by the neck after a long difficult day but this really will get you nowhere. Do not forget that they probably asked the right person who conveniently 'forgot' to do it. You will quickly establish which of your peers consistently 'forget' to complete certain tasks such as rewriting drug charts or prescribing TTA sheets, leaving it instead for the on-call doctor to do.

7 Not providing you with the relevant information about a situation when bleeping you. See below for an example.

8 Asking you to cannulate a patient in the middle of the night, but do not get a tray ready for you.

9 Sit there and eat chocolate or read a magazine at the nurses' station when you need assistance. A polite but firm request for some help normally will suffice, but if you are rude you will find that next time they will not bother to help at all (it can be a bit of a Catch 22 situation sometimes).

10 Ask you as the doctor on-call to change the non-urgent management of a patient not under your care instead of waiting until the team come on a ward round the next day.

*When I was a pre-registration house officer (PRHO) in respiratory medicine, I was bleeped near midnight to come to the ward to see one of the elderly patients. I knew the gentleman well, a very pleasant man who used to rivet the bodywork of aircraft together in the Second World War. The nurse had been going around the ward performing the routine observations on all the patients (pulse, blood pressure, temperature, etc.) and had come across this patient flushed and breathless. She related to me over the phone 'he is tachycardic and his blood pressure is up and he is really out of breath. Can you come quickly.' I asked for more information relating to the presence of chest pain, etc. but none was provided, as the questions had not been asked by the bedside. I ran up to the ward to see the patient who looked at me and said 'I don't know what all the fuss is about'. When I explained the nurse was worried as he was out of breath and his heart was pounding away he replied 'of course it is. I was having a cigarette outside the entrance and the lift wasn't working so I had to walk up the stairs!'*

There was no need for me to come to the ward at all. If the nurse had simply asked the patient some questions instead of relying purely on numbers on the chart then I would have had a peaceful night.

## Giving Instructions

Communication or lack of it is the chief cause of litigation within the NHS today. Lack of effective communication is particularly noticeable in some doctors compared to others. It is very easy to criticize, but often difficult for us to help others. Most of us find it relatively easy to talk to fellow doctors or patients, but the worst communication is usually to nursing staff or peer-level doctors when 'handing over' (I will come to this in a moment). All through medical school we are taught to converse with other doctors and with our patients in order to take histories. We are never taught how to communicate with nurses effectively and for this reason most doctors do not actually know what information nurses need to do their job.

As explained before, the overall duty of care remains with the doctor and in the event of a 'medical' error (as opposed to a 'nursing' error) the blame will focus on the doctor responsible as well as the department protocols. When a junior is giving instructions to nursing staff they will often be brought into question (particularly if the junior doctor is new to the department or lacking in proficiency). If a nurse has doubts about the quality of the instructions given she or he has every right to question the doctor and this practice prevents a large number of clinical incidents caused by newly qualified PRHOs. However, as juniors become more senior they dislike being questioned more and more. I dislike being questioned sometimes, particularly when I am sure of myself and of the instructions I have given. However, it is our responsibility to explain the reason for our instructions and in most cases educate our nursing staff to make them better nurses and make 'us' a better team. Therefore, even when tired, try not to lose your temper or be rude when questioned by nursing staff.

However, there are some occasions where there is no room for questioning and this is often during times of medical 'urgencies' and emergencies. If you find yourself in a situation where the nurses will not carry out your instructions for whatever reason (and I have been in this situation myself) then it is important to stay cool headed and call your senior to either affirm your instructions or change them.

When in charge of patients on the ward it is important that the nursing staff know how to manage the patient and when to call you if the condition of the patient changes. However, nurses may find a large portion of information that doctors need about a patient (for example specific examination findings, blood test trends, etc.) superfluous to their requirements.

Nurses need to know the following facts from doctors.

1 When to bleep you, that is if the parameters on a patient's observations change (for example systolic blood pressure drops, the pulse rate increases or oxygen saturations fall), at what point do you wish to be informed. This applies to patients on an individual basis.
2 Do you want to discuss anything with the patient's relatives if they appear on the ward?
3 Do you want to review the patient at a particular time?
4 Do you wish to inspect a wound? Wounds and dressings are a particular bone of contention between nurses and doctors. Animosity is easy to avoid by following simple rules and having some understanding of how the nursing day runs. Dressings are most often changed mid-morning following the early morning ward round. Thus, wounds can be inspected with 'permission' of the nursing staff easily on the morning round. However, if you wish to wait until the afternoon for a particular reason (for example the boss is attending the evening round) then let the allocated nurse know so that they do not change the dressing only to have to take it down again. Wound dressings can take between ten and 30 minutes to apply and should usually remain on for 48 hours or longer before changing.

> In summary, inspect wounds after asking the appropriate nurse if it is okay. Try in most cases to do this in the morning and let the nurse know if you wish to look at a wound at an unusual time.

5 Do you wish the nurses to pass a message to an allied health professional (for example physiotherapy, occupational therapy, speech and language therapy and dietetics).

## Relationships with Nursing Staff and Allied Health Professionals

Relationships between colleagues within any workplace is common, but particularly in hospitals where doctors and nurses are working in close proximity for long hours under stressful conditions. Doctors and nurses have been having more than just working relationships with each other since the beginning of time, but junior doctors are particularly susceptible to the allure of nurses. As undergraduates medical students have no sex appeal, but once qualified the field changes and can be a shock to the unsuspecting. This change can be exciting for obvious reasons, but can also have devastating consequences within the working environment. Some relationships can work well, but if the break up is not mutual it can mar working relationships with serious consequences. Enter into relationships with nursing colleagues with caution.

# 8

# Radiologists and Radiographers

## Requesting Investigations: Urgent Versus Non-urgent

Radiologists, like all specialists, can be intimidating to the junior doctor. While some are very friendly and approachable, you will find more than your fair share who are not. Ask any junior what their worst task is and they will always say having to discuss an investigation with the radiologist. This is often due to pressure from your own team asking you to organise a computed tomograph (CT) or magnetic resonance image (MRI) urgently or, not uncommonly, a scan that should have been requested a week ago but was forgotten and is now needed imminently.

A few years ago I read the following letter, which was submitted to the *British Medical Journal*. It epitomises every junior doctors' nightmare visit to the department of radiology. This purpose of this chapter is to teach you how to avoid a situation such as the one here and you will no doubt hear stories like this from your colleagues in the mess who have not read this book.

---

The houseman is in the middle of a ward round with my specialist registrar, and, since I am going past the X-ray department on my way to a ward visit, I decide to drop the MRI request in to the radiologists. All MRI requests must be discussed with a radiologist so I find myself in a darkened viewing room with a woman not much older than myself.

'Hello, I'm one of the geriatricians. I'm after an MRI of this chap's pituitary fossa.'

A frown, and her head is cocked to one side: 'He's not exactly top priority is he?'

I blink, and I become aware of my nostrils flaring – always a bad sign. Then I realise that I'm not wearing my identity badge.

The radiologist continues: 'What do you hope to achieve with this investigation?'

'A diagnosis would be nice.'

---

'Is he fit for surgery?'

'Best to have a diagnosis first don't you think?'

She half smiles, steps forward, and waves her hand six inches from my nose in a 'wakey wakey' sort of gesture. I think of Biff in the film *Back to the Future*.

'I'll give him one star priority because he's an inpatient, but people with broken necks or spinal cord compression will take priority over him.'

'That sounds perfectly reasonable.' I turn on my heel to go. Years of taking this sort of abuse have left their mark. I say nothing. I meekly take the flak. But this isn't the end. I'm called back.

'You haven't put your bleep number on this request.'

'I don't carry a bleep. I'm the consultant.'

Her jaw drops. Only the heat from her face matches the steam coming out of my ears. 'I'm sorry,' she says, 'I didn't realise.'

'That's alright. You can teach me to suck eggs any time you like.'

Stuttering apologies and embarrassed looks continue for some time afterwards, an awareness that boundaries have been stepped over, some unwritten rules broken. Yet there is no acknowledgement that she has been downright rude almost to the point of physical abuse, merely that she shouldn't have done this to a consultant colleague. She clearly thinks this sort of behaviour dished out to juniors is entirely acceptable.

A straw poll of my department's senior house officers confirms this.

So what do I do? The story makes for a good ward round anecdote, and I could leave matters there. I could be working with this radiologist for the rest of my professional life. After all, the problem on one level is merely about good manners and common courtesy. On another, however, it's about bullying in the workplace. The alternative? Bring the whole clinical governance machine to bear on the issue. The clinical director of radiology is going to return my call. …[1]

Just like everything else in medicine, if approached logically and calmly the process becomes much easier. You need to know the following information before going to discuss anything with a radiographer or radiologist and be able to present it in a concise and logical order.

1   Who – patient name, age and sex.
2   What – what type of investigation?

---

[1] The cycle of abuse goes on. *BMJ* 2002; **325**: 831.

3  When – is it an emergency or urgent or routine investigation?
4  Where – on the ward, in accident and emergency, in theatre or in the radiology department.
5  Extras – is the patient coming with any additional requirements or equipment that may make the investigation more difficult to perform? For example, are there intravenous or oxygen lines *in situ*? Is the patient critically ill and in need of a nurse and doctor escort? Is the patient mentally ill, violent or confused?
6  Concurrent illness – does the patient have significant disease of any other systems about which the radiologist needs to know, for example renal disease in a patient going for an angiogram (the contrast is subject to renal excretion and can precipitate renal failure) or an abdominal aortic aneurysm in a patient going for a biliary tree ultrasound scan?
7  Allergy – does the patient have a history of anaphylaxis or allergy?
8  How – will they get to the radiology department, on a bed or in a wheelchair or will they walk in?
9  Performer – who does your team expect to perform the investigation? Is a specific consultant or radiographer required?

Lastly, after you have supplied the information to the radiologist, if the request is accepted you then need to ask some questions of the radiologist.

1  Patient: do they need to do anything beforehand, for example nil by mouth or should they be well hydrated?
2  Doctor: do you need to do anything to the patient before, during and after the procedure, for example administer a premed, give intravenous fluids or monitor urine output?
3  Nurses: do the nurses need to do or know anything before the patient comes down?

## Radiological Procedures: What Information Is Required and What to Do

The difference between an investigation and a procedure is that one is non-invasive and one is invasive, respectively. Investigations usually require minimal input from the junior doctor and once the investigation is performed the patient goes back to the ward and needs minimal extra care. In contrast, a radiological procedure can produce significant extra work and the patient may require much more care before and after the event.

The following are just a few examples of radiological procedures.

1  Biopsy: can be ultrasound or CT guided.
2  Contrast studies: usually injected intravenously, intra-arterially or given orally, rectally, etc. Used for examining blood vessels (for example, an intra-arterial digital

subtraction angiogram (IADSA)) and the bowel (barium meal, follow-through or enema).

3 Stent deployment: introduction of a self-expanding metal stent (memory metal) or plastic stent into a tube, for example oesophagus, common bile duct and peripheral arteries.

For care of patients after radiological procedures you can follow the outlines listed above in the section on some questions to ask the radiologist, but you will need to supplement your plan of care by asking more experienced ward-based staff such as your specialist registrar (SpR) and senior nurses. The very best example of this interaction can be found on a vascular surgery ward where these types of procedures are performed on many patients on a daily basis. Often integrated care pathways are in place to make sure all patients are well monitored.

## Specialist Radiology

Traditionally the term 'specialist radiology' has been applied to most radiological investigations not using traditional methods, that is X-rays for producing radiographs. However, with the introduction of more and more technology, CT and MRI scanning has become part and parcel of everyday radiology and specialist examinations are now considered those investigations that are required to be performed by radiologists that have specialised in a particular field. Some of these investigations use radioisotopes and are performed in a separate department called nuclear medicine (also colloquially referred to as unclear medicine, usually because most doctors are unable to read the scans themselves and require a radiologist to write a report). Examples include the following.

1 Vascular: duplex, IADSA and magnetic resonance angiography.

2 Scintigraphy: contrast study using injected radionucleotides. The best example is a bone scan to determine the presence of bony metastasis from a primary tumour. Others include scintimammograms ($^{99}$Te), scintiangiography (used for determining organ function based on the distribution of the blood supply, for example a thallium scan for cardiac function), renal scanning (mercaptoacetylglycine (MAG-3), dimercaptosuccinic acid (DMSA) or diethylene triamine penta-acetic acid (DTPA)) and bone scans.

3 Positron emission tomography (PET) scanning: using radioactive particles for detecting the presence of tumour deposits. Particularly useful for looking at the mediastinum, which is inaccessible to biopsy.

Specialist radiological procedures can be tricky to organise, not because the radiologists are difficult to corner, but usually because the request forms are difficult to find unless you are based on a specialist ward. The easiest way to find forms is to go to the relevant ward and ask a staff nurse to tell you where they are kept. Make sure you introduce yourself first or are wearing hospital identification otherwise you will not be given one. If that fails then telephone the department (which may not even be located in your hospital: this is particularly true of PET) and ask their receptionist's advice. Often you may have to type out a referral and fax it to the relevant department. If you are still at a loss then telephone the senior house officer in that speciality, for example vascular, breast, etc. and ask how they do it. You may find that they offer to request it for you, as they know the system so have the details to hand. Make sure you try the other avenues first as they will be sure to ask you and will not be impressed if you have not shown initiative.

# 9

# Therapists and Professionals Allied to Medicine

For the politically correct among you, professionals allied to medicine are now called allied health professionals. This fancy title encompasses some of the most important people you will work with, who not only make a huge difference to your patients, but will make your life easier as they help to get your patients home. Often doctors, who are ignorant of what they do, do not give these highly skilled individuals the respect they really deserve. Now, as a qualified doctor I interact with them every day and notice that other doctors who ignore them are those who do not get on with nurses or their patients either. As an undergraduate I really had no concept of what these people did until I had to spend two days with them as part of my senior curriculum. Only then did I understand. If you are sociable and want to do the best for your patients then read on ...

## Physiotherapists

It was not until I injured my shoulder to the extent that I could not write or drive that I went to see the consultant orthopaedic surgeon I was under for my senior firm. He said he could not do much except inject it with steroids and referred me for physiotherapy.

To my humbling surprise, the physiotherapist's knowledge of functional anatomy was better than mine and their breadth of knowledge was impressive. My muscle spasm was released and carefully tailored exercises were given to me to strengthen the muscles I had injured. Not only did my shoulder improve, where so-called 'medical management' could do little, but the physiotherapist actually determined why I had injured my shoulder in the first place. No longer was the cause a 'beer injury', but she discovered that I had something called a muscle imbalance. This was determined by assessing my biomechanics.

It is disgraceful that the medical profession still regard physiotherapists as a bunch of masseuses/masseurs who work with hot towels and oils. Anyone with an injury who has seen a physiotherapist will tell you this is not the case. Physiotherapists will get your in-patients mobile, which decreases their complication rate and gets them home sooner. Once the patients have gone home, they are seen in the out-patient department to make sure that they stay mobile. This is to prevent and reduce further hospital admissions.

## Occupational Therapists

This is a broad speciality covering everything from hand therapy to mental health rehabilitation and back to organising hand rails and raised toilet seats for hip replacement patients. Occupational therapists are a friendly bunch whom you will come across mostly in the orthopaedic setting, but their role is much more than this. As with physiotherapists, occupational therapists specialise, just as doctors do, into an area they enjoy and can make a difference. They will take patients on 'home visits' to see if they are safe to be discharged and liaise with social workers and district nurses to give the patient the support they need to get home and stay home.

## Speech and Language Therapists

If you want to know how you swallow or talk, then speak to this lot. Anyone who has a speech problem will rave to you about how skilled speech and language therapists are. However, you will probably only come across them if your patient has a stroke and you need to have their swallowing assessed. Speech and language therapists are few and far between and you would be wise to ask one to show you how to assess swallowing early on in your house jobs so that you do not keep your patients starving unnecessarily (patients are often kept nil by mouth after a stroke until their swallowing is assessed and deemed safe). Your consultant will be very impressed if you get your patients drinking early, as it will decrease their risk of complications and get them home sooner.

## Dieticians

Probably the healthiest of the bunch, they are a wealth of information on nutritional states and diet. Their expertise really comes to light when you go onto the intensive therapy unit or high-dependency unit and see them calculating a feeding regime (either parenteral or enteral) for each patient based on their disease, past medical history, weight and age.

It is important to note that 30–50% of patients admitted to hospital are suffering from malnutrition and this leads to pressure sores, lowered immunity, decreased skeletal and cardiac muscle function and reduced cellular function to mention just a few. In surgical patients it leads to poor wound healing and increased post-operative complications. Therefore, it does not take a genius to work out that you will need to get the dietician to see half of your patients and improve their nutritional status.

The bottom line is do not underestimate the importance of all the other health professionals around you. If you do not know what they do, then it is better to ask them than to ignore them. We are all here for the same purpose – the care of our patients. Anything that you can do to improve their care should be done. Secondly, if you are clever and have read between the lines then you will realise that, as a busy pre-registration house officer/senior house officer, you can ask the expertise of others, which will take less time than trying to work all these things out on your own. Your consultant will be most impressed if the post-operative infection rates suddenly decrease because you have been improving the nutritional status of your patients or getting them mobile early.

# 10

# Referring and Requesting

Throughout all stages of your medical career you will have to refer to and accept referrals from other doctors and nurses. Unfortunately, the way of the world is that the most junior on the team is always given the job of referring, as it can be awkward, difficult and time-consuming. The practical joke of the matter is that you will always be asked to refer to a more senior doctor, but it is the junior on the team with the least experience who has to make the referral!

A large proportion of doctors, but not all, do not like to receive referrals as it involves more work for already overworked people. For this reason, doctors such as this to whom you are referring will usually find some way of refusing a referral or delaying when they need to come and see the patient. This attitude, while not necessarily in the correct ethos of medicine, is entirely understandable and should not be scoffed at without thought.

For this reason referring is perhaps one of the most difficult tasks for the junior doctor and this section has the following objectives:

- to make it easier and less stressful to refer
- to make you sound more knowledgeable
- to make you more professional
- to reduce the likelihood of your referral being refused or delayed

## Why Refer?

Throughout all stages of a clinical career it is necessary to refer patients to other specialists for their opinion. This is because our breadth of medical/surgical knowledge decreases with seniority and, conversely, depth increases. Thus, one would not expect a chest physician to know the intricacies of biliary surgery and likewise one would not expect a cardiac surgeon to know all about oncology, etc. It may be surprising to some readers (and some consultants!) to know that is it most often the case that the senior house officer/pre-registration house officer (SHO/PRHO) on a surgical firm may be better at managing a 'medical' problem than their seniors and vice versa on medical firms. However, when a ward patient is unwell it would be professionally and ethically inappropriate for a junior to manage the patient alone and therefore 'senior' specialist opinion is sought. Some juniors may disagree with this statement thinking they are able to deal with most problems. However, imagine if a close relative or parent was unwell post-operatively with a lobar pneumonia. You would want a chest physician to see them to give advice on local sensitivities or up to date British Thoracic Society guidelines rather than let the surgical SHO treat the patient using their knowledge alone, however competent they may be.

It should be noted though that, even if a referral is made, it is not always necessary for that patient to be seen by the specialist. You or your firm may be more than happy to manage the patient after seeking telephone advice, but this advice can only be given if the appropriate referral is made.

## Types of Referral

Effective and appropriate communication is the mainstay of referring. One needs to imagine the information we would require if we were listening to a referral. This information differs, depending on the type of referral, which should always be stated at the beginning (Figure 10.1).

## Refer to Whom?

The first rule of referring is to make sure you are referring to the correct speciality and then the correct firm. Let me explain: in different hospital trusts the same clinical diagnosis may not be treated/accepted by the same firm. For example, both medical and surgical firms may treat pancreatitis, while accident and emergency (A&E) consultants, general surgeons, orthopods or neurologists/neurosurgeons may manage head injuries. Most often your seniors or senior nursing staff will be able to inform you of the customs in your hospital.

Sometimes your consultant will wish you to refer a patient to a particular consultant rather than a speciality, which may consist of several consultants. (In some hospitals there is reciprocity between teams.) Most often, however, it is the consultant on-call to whom in-patients should be referred. This information is listed in A&E majors and in the switchboard each day. The referral 'for' a consultant will usually be 'taken' by his/her specialist registrar (SpR) or SHO and again your seniors or senior nursing staff will be able to inform you. If you are in doubt it is better to bleep the SHO and ask their advice: they will either take the referral or ask you to bleep their registrar.

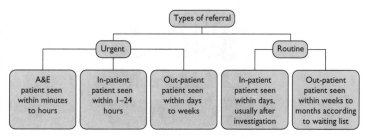

**Figure 10.1** Types of referral.

## The 'Art'

The information required is no different in bulk from that which a medical student can easily obtain from questioning and observation using common sense. The art is in the presentation.

Once you have bleeped and you are telephoned back, introduce yourself and make sure you are talking to the correct person as often a nurse or medical student may answer a bleep if the doctor is busy. It would be a waste of time for both of you to start referring to the wrong person.

Name, age, ward or clinic location and referring consultant are all obvious points but next is the presentation: what, how and when, with salient, related, past medical and surgical, drug and social history. In addition, include previous admissions with the same complaint and, if a particular consultant already knows the patient. What the relevant examination findings were at presentation, what treatment you have given and what the examination findings are now. Penultimately, include what would you like the doctor to whom you are referring the patient to do (Figure 10.2).

Lastly, how soon do you want the patient seen, expressed in minutes, hours or days. It is perfectly reasonable for a PRHO to ask an SpR to be on the ward within five minutes if your patient is 'going off', but what a registrar does not want, is to be asked to rush up to a ward to see an 'urgent' referral when in reality it could have waited six or even 24 hours.

All the information required seems commonsense and indeed it is, but when you are anxious about speaking to a more senior doctor whom you may not know, it is easy to forget to give or ask the most important details. This is particularly the case in the adrenaline rush of speaking to a senior whom you have woken up or who seems annoyed that you have bothered them.

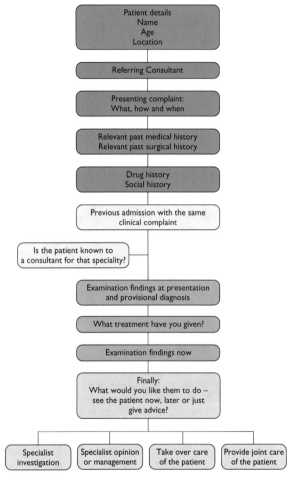

**Figure 10.2** Information required for referring a patient.

Often, if you have woken someone up, they will be half asleep too and forget to ask you important information you have forgotten to volunteer. This can have potentially disastrous consequences. The following is a witnessed case scenario.

*A year 1 medical SHO was referred a patient by a year 1 casualty SHO. The patient had presented with an acute 'asthma attack' in the early hours of the morning. The medical SHO was dealing with an unwell patient on the ward and was tired. He accepted the referral without protest and left the unwell patient on the ward for the A&E department, thinking that the patient with the asthma attack would be more unwell and therefore take priority. On arrival in the A&E department he discovered the patient sitting up talking in full sentences, having been managed through the acute phase by the A&E staff. He rapidly returned to the ward without consequence to the other patient, but cursed himself for having left the ward without asking the vital question of 'how the patient was now', not 'how were they on arrival'.*

The lesson here is that the A&E SHO did not refer the patient properly and the medical SHO did not 'take' the referral well. Effective communication failed and a patient was put in danger. When the basic things go wrong, mistakes happen. When these basic day-to-day tasks become second nature the job gets much easier, but hopefully if you have read this you will be well ahead of the game.

Accidents are the result of human error. Eternal vigilance is the price of safety.

# 11

# Clinics

## Out-patient Clinics

The general practitioner or another consultant usually refers patients. These referrals may be urgent (patient seen within two weeks) or routine (patient not usually seen within at least six to eight weeks of referral).

Out-patient clinics are run by a clinic manager (usually a senior sister or nurse who has taken on a part managerial, part clinical role). The team is expected to attend in full unless stated otherwise by your seniors. The clinic nurse(s) will provide a computer-generated list of patients that are expected to attend, identifying new patients and follow-up attendees. The consultant will usually highlight those patients to be seen by the senior and junior members of the team. Junior doctors should present their patients to the specialist registrar (SpR) or the consultant (as per the instructions of the consultant) before instigating out-patient management (obviously).

If patients are to be admitted from the clinic then they should be clerked and examined there and then. A drug and fluid chart should be completed and any blood or radiographic investigations performed in the out-patients department before the patient goes to the ward. From here you can follow the admission checklist given in Table 4.3.

## Fracture Clinics

The casualty senior house officer (SHO) or occasionally SpR refers patients directly from the accident and emergency (A&E) department. These patients have presented to the A&E department within the last few days with an acute injury. They will have a suspected or confirmed fracture that has been treated in a 'back slab' (half plaster of Paris cast which allows soft tissue swelling in the few days after a bony injury). The orthopaedic team has not usually seen these patients before.

The diagnosis is established or confirmed in the fracture clinic and further management is instigated. The patient and their fracture is either treated conservatively in plaster and followed up or admitted from the clinic for fracture fixation (that is surgery). These clinics are excellent learning opportunities in orthopaedic management.

## Pre-admission/Pre-assessment Clinics

See Chapter 4. Usually just the pre-registration house officer attends. In some specialist fields the SHO attends.

# 12

# The Operating Theatre

This is a rough guide as to what to do, who to get on side and what not to do. Being in theatre can be the most incredible experience or your worst nightmare. Aspiring surgeons can hate being on a surgical firm (as I did as an undergraduate) and, equally, career physicians or general practitioners can love their theatre time. With a little knowledge regarding the staff and general running of theatres you will find your time much more enjoyable. The golden rule is if in doubt ask, but there are other secrets to being in theatre.

## Getting to Know the Staff

The following people, who can seem unnerving at first, staff theatres.

1  A theatre sister who is in charge of the running of the theatre and will often dictate orders to you and your consultant!
2  A scrub nurse who prepares the instrument trays and assists the surgeon during the operation.
3  An anaesthetic consultant, specialist registrar (SpR) or senior house officer who will provide general or regional anaesthesia for the patient. Any procedure done under local anaesthetic does not require an anaesthetist.
4  An operating department assistant (ODA) who will provide assistance to the anaesthetic team and nurses, usually by providing equipment and setting up machines.
5  Theatre nurses – as on the ward, they make sure the care of the patient runs smoothly.
6  Nurses trained as surgical assistants – this is becoming more common and you may notice it in orthopaedics.

All of these individuals are senior and have invariably worked together for many years so know each other well. As with any circle of friends, the newcomer finds it difficult to break into the ring and should not be put off if the first few attempts fail. The first and most important thing to do when you walk into the operating theatre is to introduce yourself to all present. Make sure that the nursing staff know your name and grade, particularly the scrub nurse. You will find that the scrub nurse can be your best ally during a difficult operation and the trust and friendship that develops between you will be invaluable when you are operating alone or when on-call. I have been saved on more than one occasion by the scrub nurse, who has told me which suture type my consultant prefers for wound closure. This has allowed my consultant to gain confidence in me and prevents embarrassing ticking off sessions on the post-operative ward round.

When talking to your registrar or consultant in the first few weeks of your post, before you know them well, keep small talk to appropriate breaks in the surgeon's concentration and the subject professional at first.

## Learning Anatomy

Theatres are the place to improve your knowledge of anatomy, but not to 'learn' it. This may sound strange, but I guarantee that you will find it more productive to learn your anatomy at home before entering the operating theatre. When you are assisting you can then see the anatomy you have learnt come to life and appreciate it in three dimensions as well as see variations between individuals.

All theatre operation lists must be submitted a day in advance (except emergency lists), so that it is always possible to find out which operations are to be performed the following day. If you cannot find the list then ask your SpR. Your seniors will always question you in theatre on your anatomy and it pays to read up the night before. Do this every time and not only will you impress your boss, but you will accelerate your anatomical and surgical knowledge.

## Dos

1  Introduce yourself to nursing and anaesthetic staff.
2  Engage in conversation with your colleagues.
3  Ask sensible questions, particularly if you do not understand something: this is the only way to learn. If you feel the timing is not appropriate then wait until after the operation and then ask (I often do this – it shows maturity and an understanding that the surgeon is concentrating).
4  Offer to make coffee/tea for your seniors after a long operation (they will be as tired as you). It shows respect for your seniors.
5  Ask to perform part of an operation if you think you are able or ask to be shown how to perform it so you know for next time.
6  Ask to be taught how to write an operation note.

## Don'ts

1  Engage in conversation during emergencies.
2  Be rude to nursing staff. If you do, it will be your funeral!
3  Sulk if you are not allowed to do something. Your seniors are not out to get you and there will be a good reason that you may not understand. You are within your rights to ask for an explanation after the operation. This is actually a good way to improve your surgical understanding as long as you take the correct approach.
4  Ever walk into theatre without overshoes or theatre clogs on. This contaminates theatre floors and means that the nursing staff will have to clean them again. Making nurses do more work than necessary … bad move.
5  Ever eat or drink in theatre. See the note on shoes.
6  Ever touch instruments on the scrub trolley without the express permission of the scrub nurse.
7  Ever place your gloved hands into a wound without the express permission of the surgeon.
8  Turn your head away from the surgical field to sneeze. The purpose of a mask is to prevent droplets from your mouth from being projected forward. There are gaps at the side of the mask to let these particles out. If you turn your head to sneeze you will fire your germs straight into the wound. If you have to sneeze, then simply lean back but face forward.

# 13

# Laboratory Investigations

These constitute the vast majority of investigations junior doctors request, which include all blood tests as well and other body fluid samples testing. The following are the departments commonly dealt with by all house officers:

- haematology
- biochemistry
- microbiology
- transfusion
- virology
- histopathology

All junior doctors should have a list of the daytime and on-call telephone numbers of each of these departments which will save hours on the telephone to the switchboard in the middle of the night. Just like any other department there is a hierarchy of seniority in these departments and a consultant who works in conjunction with the chief technician usually heads each one. You can imagine that each patient in hospital has on average one blood test a day and perhaps one body fluid examination every three or four days (for example a mid-stream urine or wound swab). If the hospital has 1000 beds you can imagine how busy these departments are.

For run of the mill non-urgent investigations there is no need to discuss requests, unless you are contacted by the laboratory. They will always bleep you if there is a problem. However, if you need to request an unusual or urgent investigation then telephoning the department is not only courteous, but it will ensure that the test is actually performed. This is particularly important outside normal working hours when samples are often only picked up from the drop box (where the porters or vacuum chutes leave them) if the technician is telephoned in advance. When speaking to departments always ensure that you are talking to the relevant person at the start of the conversation and then explain your request. There is rarely any problem with requests being accepted unless it is the middle of the night where you will be asked for clinical justification. This is rarely a taxing matter however, and a simple reply usually suffices.

One small note that will win you favour is to inform the on-call technician in advance if you know that you will be taking a sample in the middle of the night. This information is invaluable as they will keep the machines running and stick around in the hospital until the sample arrives. In small hospitals the technicians often go home, as there is little work at night and only return to the hospital if bleeped by you. Saving them a journey home and back again will make their life easier and also means that you will get your result faster. Usually you will be waiting up to get the result, so you can see how a one-minute telephone call at 9 p.m. can save you a one-hour wait in the middle of the night.

# 14

# Getting Registered and Applying for Senior House Office Posts

## Clinical Tutor

At the beginning and end of each six-month post (or four-month post if you are doing a 3 × 4) you will be assessed by your clinical tutor. This person is usually but may not always be your consultant. You will be introduced to them in the first week of your post (supposedly), but quite often the time you start a job is when they are away on holiday. It is best to meet them for your first appointment as early as possible. It is your responsibility to get in touch with them. During your 'interview', which is more like an informal chat, you will be asked what your expectations of the post are and what your career plans are (if you have any). You will also be asked whether you have any queries or worries. If you have any professional or personal problems that may interfere or are interfering with your job you should discuss them with your tutor. Your tutor will be surprisingly understanding and is there to help you rather than to intimidate or hinder you. The purpose of this meeting is not only for you to find out what is expected of you, but also for the department to find out what you expect of them. It may sound unusual that you can have expectations, but if you are in a training post then the trust and department has an obligation to provide ward- and lecture-based 'bleep-free' teaching, as well as practical on-the-job training. Often departments and trusts do not provide the required teaching and it is not unreasonable to make a complaint about this early on in your post to your clinical tutor. With decreasing hours on the job it is important to get the most out of your training.

## General Medical Council Registration

It is surprisingly easy to get full registration and here is why: the government has spent in excess of £150 000 to train you over a period of five to six years depending on your course. They want to register you because they need a return on their investment. It is actually quite difficult not to get registered. In fact your salary as a pre-registration house officer (PRHO) is paid not by your hospital, but by your medical school and the hospital is paid to take you on. What this means is that, as a PRHO, you are there to learn and not just provide a service for the hospital.[1] There are various political reasons including this conspiring to make sure you get registered. This does not mean that you should sit on your backside and be lazy. On the contrary, most consultants will pick up on who is a good or bad PRHO very quickly and make a note of things for your reference. The efforts you put in as a PRHO will ultimately get you a good reference and provide you with the knowledge that will get you into a good senior house officer (SHO) post.

Once you are into your second house job you will need to start thinking about which SHO/F2 posts to apply for. At this stage, once you have decided on a basic career path (that is medicine, surgery, general practice, obstetrics and gynaecology, etc.), you have two options: rotation or stand alones?

## Rotations

These are a series of six-month posts linked to one hospital, but usually based at several hospitals within close proximity. There is an SHO for each hospital post and at the end of each six months all SHOs rotate until each has spent six months in each post. When you apply for a rotation you are applying for all of these posts in one go.

Rotations may last between 18 months (three posts) and three years (six posts). The three-year posts take you through the first sets of postgraduate examinations (parts 1 & 2 and 3) and can lead directly to a specialist registrar (SpR) post. Rotations are based within a region when outside London (for example East Anglia or Yorkshire) or within a section of London (north east London). Rotations are a good choice if you wish to settle down in one region for a period of time, but there are a few drawbacks. You may have to rotate into a post you do not wish to do (for example urology, ear, nose and throat, etc.) or rotate into a hospital that you do not like. All rotations have excellent posts, mediocre posts and one or two posts that are not liked. Rotations are good as you need not worry about the hassle of applying for jobs and interviews every six months, but they do tie you down for the duration of the rotation. It is becoming increasingly common for SHOs to organise themselves to do the post they least like at the end of the rotation. This then leaves the option of dropping out of the

---

[1] This changes as an SHO, as the postgraduate deanery pays 50% of your salary and the hospital itself pays 50%, which means that your role as an SHO is 50% learning and 50% service provider.

rotation six months early (this does not have a detrimental effect on your career if planned early).

## Stand Alones

These posts are, as they sound, single six-month posts that you must apply for individually. They have the benefit that you can apply for posts you would like to do in hospitals you wish to work in. However, each post must be applied for, four to six months in advance, so once into a post you must immediately start thinking about the next one. If you like moving around or want to tailor your rotation then stand alones are perfect for you.

I should point out I have chosen the path of stand alone posts as I wanted to take a year out for sports and to travel. In the last 12 months, the number of stand alones has decreased considerably as they have been absorbed into rotations and F2 year programmes. It is my suspicion that the number of stand alones will gradually decline over the next few years making it more and more difficult to complete your training this way.

The upside to this is that interview panels are becoming increasingly aware that junior doctors wish to take time out of their training to pursue other avenues that life has to offer. It is therefore becoming easier to take time out within a rotation (that is complete one year, then have a year off and defer the rest of the rotation), but this question should be raised at interview if you are thinking about it.

## Location

Once you have decided which type of post you want you need to decide on your location: London or outside London?

Many juniors, particularly those who graduate from London schools, have the false belief that if you want to end up in London as a consultant then you must do all your training in London 'to get your foot in the door'. This is not strictly true although there is a significant 'old boy' network and culture, which some would say is in decline. I would say that it is simply becoming more covert.

The bottom line is that, if you are proficient in your work, good humoured, enthusiastic and diligent, then you will be able to get a job anywhere at any time. It is certainly true that, as an SpR, you will find it easier to get a consultant post in the region in which you have been an SpR. This is not necessarily the case for an SHO. However, to add complications to my previous statement, it is also easier to get your SpR number in the area in which you have done your senior SHO training as, at this stage in your career, many things work by word of mouth. It is often that 'who you know' not 'what you know' comes true.

## Where Is the Dole Office?

The next few years will cause serious employment difficulties for SHOs. At the time of writing 1 in 3 PRHOs finishing their PRHO year have no SHO training post to go to. Many have been forced to locum and others are going abroad. I know of at least 3 doctors from my hospital who cannot get an SHO post so have decided to move to Australia (2 are so fed up that they are emigrating). At present doctors applying for SHO training posts in medicine will send off on average 112 applications before obtaining a post and the average number of applicants per post is about 150.[2] The picture for surgery is not dissimilar. The next few years while the Foundation Scheme is being phased in are going to be difficult for those desperately trying to obtain posts as it is my understanding that the number of doctors exceeds the number of posts available. Inevitably some of you will be forced into Trust grade posts or locum work, but I would strongly advise you not to be disheartened as you will certainly not be alone. Patience and an ear-to-the-ground will be required but if you do find yourself unemployed, make the most of that time. See the section on taking time off. You could gain experience overseas, perform voluntary work (it doesn't help with paying off those student loans though) or gain new skills. Whatever you do, make sure that you keep applying for posts well in advance and have at least 2 SHOs and 2 SpRs look at your CV. Consultants can be very useful but you have to pick the right one, as some are happy to say that every detail is fine when in reality your CV needs a revamp. Juniors and middle grades are more likely to spend time giving you an honest opinion.

[2] Royal College of Physicians Junior Posts Competition.

# 15

# Getting on in Your Senior House Officer Post

## What Is Expected of You

Now that you have completed your pre-registration year you should have hopefully seen most of the common medical and surgical emergencies and know how to treat or have treated a large proportion of them. Some of you may have performed minor surgical procedures either in the operating theatre or in the accident and emergency (A&E) department. All new senior house officers (SHOs) should be competent in basic ward-based practical procedures, for example pleural taps, chest drain insertions, arterial blood gas, etc.

As an SHO you have already started down the road to specialisation by deciding on general practice, medicine or surgery. The majority of you will be on a rotation that will lead to becoming a specialist registrar (SpR). As such, you are expected to be far more dedicated and enthusiastic in your work, as well as more proficient than when you were a PRHO/FY1. This is a daunting situation to be thrown into overnight, from being a PRHO/FY1 to SHO/FY2. In this respect taking an A&E post in your first six months as an SHO is highly advisable to bridge the transition, as it encourages development of diagnostic skills, how to cope with life-threatening situations and practical procedures.

As an SHO you are expected to be a fully integrated (that is a working part of your team) and functional individual (that is able to perform tasks as opposed to just being there for training purposes). As such, you will be taught how to see and manage patients on your own in order to aid the smooth running of the firm. However, you will also be taught your own limitations and when to call more senior members for advice. You will be taught in the out-patients department as well as on the ward. If applicable, you will be taught in the operating theatre. See below for further details.

### Out-patient Departments

You will usually see a mixture of follow-up and new patients. By the end of each post you will be expected to manage and, in some cases, discharge follow-ups at your consultant's instruction as well as see, diagnose and formulate a treatment/investigation plan for new attendees. At the beginning of each post you will be expected to present all patients to either your SpR or consultant.

### Wards

This is where you will spend the majority of your time if you do not have a PRHO. However, it is also where you will receive most of your teaching. By the end of your post you will be able to manage the ward more or less on your own, discussing any complex issues with your SpR. If you have a houseman you will be expected to give teaching and guidance to them in a professional and caring manner. It is no longer acceptable to give all the dross jobs to the house officer. However, there are always some dull jobs the SHO has to delegate.

### Theatres

Your consultant (mainly) and your SpR should teach you how to assist in a competent manner (however, it is often the SpR who does most of the teaching). You will have picked up some skills and insight as a medical student and PRHO, but this is the time when you really learn how to assist. As an SHO you will be taught the techniques and intricacies of each operation and this will give you an understanding of how a surgeon needs assistance and when. When you are deemed competent in assisting you are more than likely to be shown how to perform surgical tasks and minor procedures. It is strongly recommended that you undertake a basic surgical skills course as early on as possible in your SHO training. It is mandatory to take this course before entering your membership examination.

Once you have passed Member of the Royal College of Surgeons parts 1 & 2 (the multiple choice questions) then you will be allowed to operate more freely than before and surgeons will be more willing to teach you. The underlying reason for this has yet to be explained but presumably stems from the initiation into the 'surgeon's club' once you have your first Royal College qualification!

## Writing Police Statements

Police statements can be exciting at first, but soon become tiresome when you are handed cases by the basket. Anyone who has worked in the A&E department will tell you the same story. However, although sometimes a chore, these statements often form the backbone of legal cases and should be written in the most professional and organised manner possible. On the whole, most barristers do not twist medical statements or squeeze medical professionals into corners in court, but it only takes one carelessly written statement or a single wrong fact to put you into a corner, which is unpleasant (to say the least). Speaking from experience, having written a statement in the middle of a quiet night shift in the A&E department and sent it off, all seemed well. That was until I was summoned to court and realised that I had not written my statement in exactly the same format that I remembered because I had forgotten to keep a photocopy of it.

The following is the accepted standard format for writing a statement for a casualty officer (A&E department SHO). Ward-based reports include the same information in a slightly different fashion and you should ask your seniors for advice. You should not use any abbreviations in a statement however well recognised they are. As an SHO you will be called as an actual witness not an expert witness and, therefore, in your statement you should give fact only and not opinion (see the section on going to court). Opinions lead to errors and the reputation of you and your department can be damaged.

## Format for Writing Police Statements (from the Accident and Emergency Department)

I, (name), have the following qualifications: (include your degree(s) and post-graduate examinations if any). On (date) at (time) I was on duty as a (grade and speciality) in the (department) of (hospital with address).

At (time) I saw (name of patient) who was brought into the department by (mode of transport, for example ambulance or wheelchair), having allegedly been assaulted/involved in a road traffic accident/attempted suicide, etc.

The attending paramedic/police officer stated ... Give the details given to you by the paramedics/police or any eye witnesses on the scene about the pre-hospital events which you know to be true. Particular details on the mechanism of any injury may be appropriate (for example damage to vehicles), but do not speculate.

The patient told me ... Give details of the history the patient gave you, writing the patients own words in inverted commas if possible.

My immediate or life-saving treatment was ... (for example oxygen, intravenous cannula and fluids). Follow this with your examination findings.

I requested the following investigations (list the investigations requested) and they showed (their results). A diagnosis of (list) was made.

Further treatment was necessary (for example mobilisation and stabilisation of a fracture, chest drain, etc.). This was administered by ...

The patient was discharged/referred to (give the speciality) at (time). The patient was seen by (Doctor X, grade and speciality) at (time).

Note: surprisingly often the police do not take detailed statements from admitting teams, so it is worth adding a note of the outcome of the patient. For example, at (time) Doctor X, the orthopaedic senior house officer saw Mr Smith. He was seen by the orthopaedic specialist registrar at (time) and transferred to the operating theatre for surgical fixation of (injury). After theatre he was admitted to a surgical ward. In these final details it may be necessary to be vague if you are unsure of the admission details. It is acceptable to state that the patient was admitted under the care of the on-call team (stating speciality).

At the end of your statement you should write 'End of statement' and sign it.

## Going to Court

If you have written a police statement then you may, several months later, be summoned to appear in court and give evidence relating to your statement. You may be asked for a further statement a few weeks before attending court in which you will be asked to give your opinion by a member of the Criminal Investigation Department. Unfortunately, police officers are not educated how the medical hierarchy system works and do not think it unreasonable that a doctor two or three years out of medical school give their expert opinion.

> As a junior, when you attend court, it will be as an 'actual witness'. This means that you have had first-hand contact with a patient and you are called to give the facts of your encounter only. No suppositions, inferences or opinions should be sought or given. This is the golden rule.

Suppositions, inferences and opinions are the task of the expert witness who is usually a consultant or SpR. If you are asked to give your opinion, as I have been, you should refuse, but it is easier said than done.

If you are ever asked to give an opinion you should discuss it with your consultant or, in the A&E department, the head of department. A&E departments are well experienced in dealing with court cases and statements. Usually a single consultant will vet any statement that is to leave their department and, if you are summoned to court, they will attend with you for moral support. However, the problem arises when you are called to attend after you have left the post. In this case, you should still contact your old head of department for advice.

Another trick played when you arrive at court is for the barrister leading the case to go over your statement with you and hint that you will have to give your opinion when you are on the stand. Again, do not do this when you are attending as an actual witness.

Taking the stand and giving evidence providing you stick to the golden rule is surprisingly easy and should not be a nerve-wracking experience. You will be called into the courtroom and asked to swear in using a holy book of your choice (Bible, Torah, Koran, etc.). If you are agnostic you swear in by other means. Once you are on the stand you will face the jury (if there is one) and the barristers. The judge is usually to your side.

Everyone in the courtroom is there at that point to hear what you have to say. They are not there to harass or belittle you. They will ask you only simple questions (providing you stick to the golden rule) and expect straightforward answers. If you feel that you are being harassed then you may ask for the judge to intervene, but usually he or she will do this before you need to. Doctors are respected in court and are treated well. So do not be afraid. If at any point you feel unwell you may ask for a chair or some water. Once you have given your evidence you must remain on the stand until the judge has given you permission to leave.

Once you have left the stand you are usually allowed to go home or permitted to sit in the public gallery to hear the remainder of the case. The Witness Service will give you a form for claiming your expenses, whereby you can claim for your time and travelling expenses. This form can be completed when you get home and posted. A cheque for a significant sum in your favour usually arrives within two weeks, but this extra source of income should be declared to the tax man!

## When Patients Are Mismanaged

This section applies more to SHOs, as they have enough experience to know when a patient has not been managed appropriately, but if you are switched on in your PRHO post then read on.

If you think that a patient has been mismanaged by other doctors or nursing staff then you need to consider one thing before getting agitated. Is the patient in danger or at risk. If so, adjust their management accordingly in a logical calm manner and explain to the nurses looking after the patient why you have changed their management.

Once the patient is safe, then consider this: if you were in the place of the person whom you feel has mismanaged the patient, what would you have done differently? It is usually best to assess this when you are relaxed and calm, often several hours or days after the event. If you still feel strongly then do not get anxious. Patients are mismanaged all the time, both in hospitals and the community, due to lack of time, experience or skill. Most commonly the errors are very minor and the patient is never in real danger.

It is natural for you to get angry and feel aggrieved, as you would not want your friends or relatives to be mismanaged. However, making a song and dance about things to chastise the person involved will not help them or the patient. Firstly, speak to the person involved and ask them politely to justify their management approach. They may have a perfectly valid reason of which you are unaware. If this does not help, then firstly discuss the matter with your peers, then with your seniors and, finally, your consultant. At this time it would be appropriate to fill in an incident report form, which will be available from the ward, which is then sent on to management.

If you still feel the matter has not been handled appropriately then you must now speak to the management staff. You must be prepared to inform your consultant and the senior nursing staff that you are doing this, as you will generate large waves. The problem now multiplies in that senior medical staff will notice your name and you need to be careful that you do not get a reputation as a troublemaker.

If you feel out of your depth then either ask your consultant to take it further or seek an independent outside opinion, which can be done anonymously.

From my experience of working at several different hospitals these matters are dealt with very differently from place to place. Some hospitals are very keen on re-educating staff and improving policy, but sadly some other trusts adopt a 'sweep it under the carpet' approach. This dangerous and downright negligent attitude usually spreads from the head of department and senior nursing staff down. Fortunately, in a department like that you will always find someone else, either medical or nursing, who is of the same mindset as you and they can be a valuable ally.

## Locum Posts

Medical temping is commonplace in fields other than doctoring. In fact, it is difficult to find a single occupational therapist, physiotherapist or nurse who does not work as a locum or bank staff member (a locum within a single National Health Service trust only) at some point in their career. Locum doctors (also known as Larry, as in Larry the locum) are becoming more common. With the government and public demanding more doctors and the European Work Time Directive decreasing the amount of hours training staff can work, the chasm of vacant doctor posts has to be filled with trust grade and locum doctors.

Locums have always had a bad reputation and are often seen as 'less capable' or 'less intelligent'. Thankfully this somewhat unfair ethos is decreasing as more training doctors do the occasional locum job on the side to supplement their income. With the changes in pay banding of most posts down to band 2B we are all losing our income. When saving for a deposit on a property or a holiday, locum work can work well in your favour.

Obtaining locums within your own hospital is extremely easy to organise and financially easier than looking outside your trust. The easiest way to do this is to give your details to the secretary organising locum work for your department or, alternatively, for locums in other specialities, visit the medical staffing department and give your details to the 'recruitment manager' organising locum work. If you are already on the payroll then your fee will simply be added to your monthly salary and tax deducted accordingly. This process is known as 'internal locuming' and is much preferred by the trust, as you will know the hospital and how it runs.

Working as a locum in a trust in which you are not employed is known as 'external locuming'. This is not difficult to arrange, but it can be more difficult to do the job as you may not know the hospital and its staff. Finding jobs is best done through a locum agency of which there are many. If you ask ten of your colleagues they will give you ten different recommendations! The agency will, of course, take their finders fee out of your pay, so you will find that you get paid less as an external locum.

# 16

## Postgraduate Examinations: Member of the Royal College of Surgeons/Member of the Royal College of Physicians

### Study Leave

This may be taken for three purposes only:

- a medical course
- a medical examination
- private study towards a medical examination

Private study is usually limited to 14 days in any six-month period and there are limitations on the amount of private study allowed depending on your trust. However, it is strongly advisable to book study leave at least six weeks in advance or longer if it is for an examination. It is common for senior house officers (SHOs) to book study leave up to three months in advance for examinations and the week before examinations to study in order to ensure they get the dates they wish.

All study leave is booked through the postgraduate centre and there is a form you must fill out that has a carbon copy, which is sent to your consultant. It is polite and professional to write a letter to your consultant asking their permission for you to take study leave in advance, as they will have to arrange cover for your on-call duties. In some trusts this is mandatory.

## Examination Structure

### Surgery

1 Part 1: a multiple choice question (MCQ) core paper covering basic surgical applied sciences of peri-operative management, trauma and critical care.
2 Part 2: an MCQ systems paper on surgical specialities, covering the anatomy, pathophysiology, investigation and treatment of disease.
3 Part 3: this is currently divided into three sections, the viva, clinical and communication skills sections, which are notoriously difficult to pass. It covers all surgical specialities in depth with knowledge of pathology and physiology expected. The viva section is divided into three stations:

- station 1: anatomy (applied surgical anatomy and operative surgery)
- station 2: physiology (applied physiology and critical care)
- station 3: pathology (applied surgical pathology and principles of surgery)

The clinical section is divided into four bays for clinical examination:

- head and neck, breast/axilla and skin
- trunk, groin and scrotum
- vascular
- orthopaedic

The communication skills section is as it sounds and does not warrant further explanation.

### Medicine

1 Part 1: two MCQ papers, both equally weighted and not negatively marked. The papers cover all medical specialities and clinical pharmacology. Candidates are only eligible after completing their first SHO post.
2 Part 2: the current part 2 is an MCQ paper with 100 non-negatively marked questions. However, the format is changing to a written examination consisting of three papers from December 2005. See the Royal College website for updates.
3 Part 3: a clinical examination (Practical Assessment of Clinical Examination Skills or PACES) currently composed of five stations, three of which are clinical stations, one is a communication skills station and the last is a verbal non-patient clinical station. The stations are as follows.

- station 1: respiratory and abdominal system examination
- station 2: history-taking skills

- station 3: cardiovascular and central nervous system examination
- station 4: communication skills and ethics
- station 5: skin/locomotor/endocrine/eye examination

## Courses

Courses are part and parcel of being an SHO, regardless of which specialty you have chosen. This section briefly outlines each course and when to apply for it.

### Surgery

1 Basic surgical skills: a workshop-based course that lasts for two to three days. It covers suturing, abdominal, bowel, vascular, orthopaedic and laparoscopic surgical techniques. Ideally it should be undertaken as early as possible in your career. This is a mandatory requirement for sitting the Member of the Royal College of Surgeons (MRCS) part 3. See the Royal College of Surgeons (RCS) website link: http://www.rcseng.ac.uk/education/courses/basic_surgical_skills.html

2 Advanced trauma life support (ATLS): a practical and theoretical course based on the American system of triage and treatment for traumatic injuries. It is usual practice to do this course alongside an accident and emergency post, but is recommended within 12 months of becoming an SHO. The course lasts for three days and is completed by sitting an examination. The examination must be passed to pass the course. If you get very high marks you may be asked to return as an instructor. This is a mandatory requirement for sitting the MRCS part 3. See the RCS website link: http://www.rcseng.ac.uk/education/courses/trauma_life_support_advanced.html

3 MRCS parts 1 & 2: several companies that are not affiliated to the RCS run courses. The majority of SHOs attend the PasTest course, which is either a weekend or five-day course depending on the size of your wallet. The five-day course is far better and more comprehensive. See the PasTest website link: http://www.pastest.co.uk/

4 Care of the critically ill surgical patient: this is aimed at more senior SHOs who have already gained the ATLS and MRCS parts 1 & 2. It covers the intensive and critical care aspect of surgery with both theoretical and practical knowledge. This is useful for a career in anaesthesia, an intensive therapy unit or trauma surgery (that is orthopaedics or general). See the RCS website link: http://www.rcseng.ac.uk/education/courses/care_of_critically_ill.html

### Medicine

1 Advanced life support: a practical- and theory-based course based on the Resuscitation Council guidelines. It is advised that this course be done in the first SHO

post in order to allow competent practice while on the crash team. This is not a mandatory requirement for sitting the Member of the Royal College of Physicians (MRCP) examination, but few SHOs would do without it.

2 MRCP: several different companies offer courses for all aspects of the examination. PasTest courses come recommended, as they do in surgery, but it is usually best to ask around your colleagues for the inside information.

# 17

# Clinical Governance

Clinical governance is a term batted around most medical schools and hospitals as job interviews approach, but does anyone really know what it means or where it came from? The important thing to note is that the principle is not a new one and what is now called clinical governance has been practised by scrupulous doctors for many years if not centuries.

Clinical governance was described in 1999 as

a framework through which NHS [National Health Service] organisations are accountable for continuously improving the quality of their services and safeguarding high standards of care by creating an environment in which excellence in clinical care will flourish.[1]

However, the standard of care depends not only on the organisation but also the individuals working within it. So further to this, the Royal College of Physicians defined it as the

acceptance of the responsibility of individual physicians to work in a way which is consistent with the values and strategic objectives of the organisation in which they are employed. Within this there is a responsibility to maintain good medical practice .... The responsibility of the organisation (Trust) is to provide appropriate facilities ... and to support the professional development ... on a continual basis.[2]

What this means is that there are two perspectives from which to view clinical governance: those of the trust and the doctor (Tables 17.1 and 17.2).

The trouble with all governmental policy is that there is always more, even when you think you have covered it all. The seven pillars of clinical governance outline the tasks each department within a trust must undertake (Table 17.3).

---

[1] Department of Health. *Health Service Circular 1999/065: Clinical Governance in the New NHS*, paragraph 6. 1999.
[2] *Physicians Maintaining Good Medical Practice: Clinical Governance and Self-regulation*. Royal College Of Physicians; 2000 (www.rcplondon.ac.uk/news/news_clin_gov.htm).

**Table 17.1** Main duties of the trust

Provide the appropriate environment and equipment
Provide the appropriate training and education (for example continuing professional development)[a]
Provide the appropriate type and number of staff[a]
Provide information for staff and patients[a]
Be accountable for care through the chief executive
Produce annual reports on governance and care
Implement National Institute of Clinical Excellence and National Service Framework guidelines[a]
Govern access to patient information as set in the Caldicott Report
Be accountable for errors

[a] Part of the seven pillars of clinical governance.

**Table 17.2** Main duties of the physician

Keep up to date with skills and training
Clinical audit[a]
Clinical research[a]
Adequate documentation[a]
Follow trust policy and national guidelines
Practise evidence-based medicine
Govern access to patient information as set in the Caldicott Report

[a] Part of the seven pillars of clinical governance.

**Table 17.3** The seven pillars of clinical governance

Clinical audit
Clinical effectiveness
Risk management
Continuing professional development and education
Research and development
Patient issues
Quality indicators: waiting times, etc.

It is clear to see that clinical governance is not an easy thing to define and often for the purposes of interviews you may be asked how clinical governance affects you in your day-to-day life: You can address this question by covering the following topics in your own words.

- documentation
- bleep-free teaching (if you actually get it)
- teaching ward rounds or firm seminars, for example a journal club
- audit and research
- postgraduate qualifications and examinations
- risk management, for example incident reporting and morbidity meetings
- full shift rotas and adequate communication in hand-over periods

# 18

# Audit

Audit, from the Latin *audire* meaning 'to hear', is defined as an official systematic examination.[1] In medicine, it is a collection of data that allows a physician to be accountable for his or her practice. Audit itself is the action of collecting the figures, which alone is simply a pointless exercise. Unless the figures are reviewed and compared to others and then acted upon patient care will not improve. This is the purpose of the 'audit cycle'.

## The Audit Cycle

The audit cycle involves observation of current practice and the setting of standards. The disparity between current practice and set standards is measured, followed by instigation and implementation of change. This must then be reassessed (audited) to check that care has improved (Figure 18.1).

All senior house officers are expected to undertake some form of audit and it is becoming more common for pre-registration house officers to perform some audit during their year. It is easy to get involved with the auditing programme and you should speak with your consultant early on in your post. Ideally you should do this within the first few weeks, as it takes a good four months to actually collect and reflect upon any good audit data. It requires considerable time for processing and is ideal if you are on a rotation and plan to stay in one hospital for 12 months or more. The most important point is that your audit idea should be original and have a purpose. There is no point conducting an audit for the sake of it, as it is very dull and time-consuming. Your audit should have a high impact on patient care and show that care in your department can be improved, particularly using new evidence.

---

[1] *Oxford English Dictionary*. Oxford: Oxford University Press; 1973.

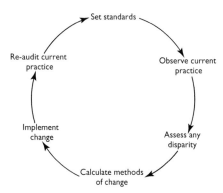

**Figure 18.1** The audit cycle.

One important point is that all information collected during the audit cycle should be anonymous or only have patient data that are necessary. The patient data should be kept secure and not available to those who do not need to see it. The data should be destroyed when it is no longer required. The Caldicott Report outlines the National Health Service policy on the handling of patient information and should be read by anyone participating in an audit: www.dh.gov.uk/PublicationsAndStatistics (Enter 'Caldicott Report' into search bar).

# 19

# A Break from the Norm...

Organisation is the key to success when taking any unpaid time off work. Generally it is not the done thing in hospital medicine, particularly in surgery, but it can be achieved, as I have done it myself. Many juniors wish to take time off at some stage in their career to travel or for personal reasons. Unfortunately, an air of egocentricism exists, which engraves in our mind that, to do so, would either make us poor doctors or ruin our careers forever. This is not always the case, but if done incorrectly it can certainly count against you in the long term. However, there are ways of making it count towards you, which I will try and convey here.

The most important item regarding time away is justification. Not only must you be able to justify this to yourself but also to your peers who will question you. Your present and all future consultants will also interrogate you. One must remember that taking time off work is an alien concept to nearly all current consultants, who have worked year after year, dedicating their lives to the National Health Service. For some of them taking time off is blasphemous. This should not stop you as, in the long run, having time away can actually make you a far better and more balanced doctor, who, on their return, is more enthusiastic, able to concentrate longer, absorb and assimilate information more quickly and so on.

I will not delve into valid reasons for taking a break, but each of you interested in doing so must produce a reason that, when questioned, will justify your absence. This sounds harsh, but is a reality in a competitive working environment. By far the single best goal you can achieve before you leave is to organise a post for your return in advance. This will successfully continue your path to further training and specialisation. This is again notoriously difficult and I was laughed at heavily when I suggested to my peers that this was my intention. However, when I achieved this both my bosses and peers were not only surprised but also proud of what I had achieved. In their eyes I had achieved the impossible – obtaining a post in one of the most competitive units in London before taking a year off to travel the world. I managed to do this by setting myself a list of goals approximately two years before leaving, the aim of which was to be at the same academic level as my peers when I returned instead of six or 12 months behind them. This meant that my curriculum vitae (CV) shone brightly before an interview and my skills of persuasion were employed at the interview. Here is my list of goals.

### Collegiate Examinations
Depending on which stage of training you are at it is important to be completely up to date if not ahead of your peers with regard to postgraduate examinations, that is if you are a new senior house officer (SHO) you should sit parts 1 & 2 as soon as possible and make sure you pass first time. This may mean spending more money on revision courses and books than your peers, but it is well worth it. If you are a senior SHO then part 3 is the obvious choice.

### Course Examinations
Make sure you have taken and passed the relevant obligatory course examinations for your stage in training, for example advanced trauma life support, advanced life support, care of the critically ill surgical patient and basic surgical skills.

### Research
By year 2 of SHO training most will probably have written up a case report, but are unlikely to have done any further research work. If you can discuss research possibilities with your consultant at the start of your SHO training then it may be possible to assist in the production of abstracts and occasionally even papers. If you can get any of your work published it will add its weight in gold to your CV. Just two published abstracts will be noted heavily at interview.

### Audit
This is another time-consuming but valuable asset. Audit is part of clinical governance and as such must be undertaken by every SHO at some stage in their training. Getting some audit experience early will give you a better understanding of clinical governance and allow you to converse at a more mature level in an interview.

### Presentation Skills
This is a simple but valuable tool in medicine. Practice makes perfect, but specialist registrars (SpRs) usually make the best tutors as they are up to date with modern technology and are used to presenting under pressure. Try to present at as many departmental and inter-departmental meetings as possible, whether it be a simple case report or research material. For each presentation for which you have compiled

the material yourself (that is a short research piece, not a patient presentation) you may add this into your CV. All these small points add up in the long run.

## Taking Time Off: Applying for Deferred Entry

Once you have achieved all or some of the above you will need to apply for posts for your return. Keep your options open by having a number of jobs at different hospitals in mind. When applying always include a covering letter. However, human resources are notoriously bad at passing these letters on to individual consultants, as I have learnt from my own experience. My advice would be to send your covering letter and a copy of your CV directly to each consultant involved as well as your completed application pack to human resources. This way when you attend for an interview the fact that you are applying for deferred entry is not a complete surprise to everyone in the room except you and the human resources person.

## Taking Time Off: Before You Go

While you are away you will need to perform certain tasks to ensure a smooth transition back into your training programme upon your return.

### Confirm the Post

Take the e-mail address of the human resources person in charge of your contract with you. E-mail them at least twice while you are away to confirm that you have accepted the position and give your return date. E-mail them again one month before your return with the same information. This will prevent human resources conveniently forgetting about you and employing another SHO in your place. I have seen this happen and the result is disastrous.

### Courses

Note down details of the courses you wish to attend on your return. This can be done before or while you are away (on-line). Have all the information necessary to apply for those courses with you. You need to apply for most courses at least three to six months in advance in my experience. The details required are your General Medical Council number, clinical tutor name and address, medical indemnity number, Royal College number, etc., as well as online banking or someone in the UK who can write a cheque for you.

### Indemnity

If you are planning to undertake medical work while away then make sure that you are covered.

*Vaccinations*
While everyone needs vaccinations for most foreign destinations doctors are at the advantage that some come at discounted prices if booked through occupational health. However, most occupational health departments run travel clinics only once a week and getting all your vaccinations make take up to two months to complete. Therefore, organise them well in advance, as you will find it very difficult and extremely costly to get immunised abroad.

## An Unusual Career

As with most things that are slightly to the side of mainstream it is often best to speak to those who move in the right channels. From my limited experience and that of my friends this is what I know and can pass on. I would thoroughly recommend speaking to those who are there to get specific information, but this should whet your appetite.

*Helicopter Emergency Medicine Service*
Not the Automobile Association, but what I would call the real 'fourth emergency service'. This is probably the most well known of the other emergency services (for example the coastguard, etc.). For those who like using ketamine on their patients and enjoy front-line hardcore trauma situations this is a fantastic career. Having had friends who have spent a year training with HEMS I can assure you that it is not for the faint of heart. It is exhilarating and you will save lives. See their website for more information: http://www.hems-london.org.uk

*Mountain Rescue*
A fantastic adjunct to a surgical career providing you are working in a mountainous region. Lesser known is the Association of Lowland Search & Rescue, which operates on the same principle as the Mountain Rescue service except in low-lying marshy areas such as Norfolk and Essex.

The training is time-consuming, but there are many different organisations that come under the umbrella of the Mountain Rescue Council. See their websites for further information about training and time commitments: http://www.mountainrescue.org.uk and http://www.alsar.org.uk/index.php

*Military*
You may find that civvy street is too dull for you. If this is the case then a career in the military seems a sensible alternative to offer you the best of both worlds – excitement, travel and medicine. Excellent careers are available for physicians and surgeons in the Royal Army, Royal Navy and Royal Air Force. See their medical web pages for further information: http://www.army.mod.uk/medical/royal_army_medical_corps/index.htm,

http://www.rafcareers.com/jobs/job_files/jobfile_medicalofficer.cfm and http://www. royal-navy.mod.uk/static/pages/3355.html

### Overseas Work

Perhaps the military is not what you had in mind, but the travel and challenge of medicine abroad excites you. There are many non-governmental organisations (NGOs) that are desperate for well-trained but senior doctors. Most of the larger organisations, such as the Red Cross and Médecins Sans Frontières (MSF), prefer to take doctors who have passed their membership examinations or those who are already SpRs. However, it is worth enquiring if you are keen to do this sort of thing. At the very least they will recommend another organisation to turn to.

MSF have an excellent website with a section devoted to doctors with their stories (physicians, surgeons and anaesthetists). Click on the 'Working for MSF' link. There is also a good page for medical students to help plan electives under 'Working for MSF' then 'Medical Students': http://www.uk2.msf.org/working4us/medicalstudents.htm

Voluntary Service Overseas is one NGO that will take on SHOs, although a basic requirement is post-qualification experience of 24 months. Like all other organisations they have opportunities as well as a need for all types of doctor. At this relatively junior level those with an interest in general and family medicine or public health will be able to offer more than a surgical SHO who does not have the experience to be able to operate independently. Check out this address: http://www.vso.org.uk/ volunteering/stepone/doctor.asp

### Sports Doctoring

The idea of being a doctor to the top teams in the world has its appeal, particularly for the sports minded. Indeed, if you ask any orthopaedic SpR about it, they will probably tell you that they are the appointed surgeon to their local rugby or football team. This is usually a good starting point, but for those who wish to take things further and want to become a registered sports doctor read on.

The field of sports and exercise medicine (SEM) is growing and currently awaiting approval from the Royal College of Surgeons (RCS) for a Certificate of Surgical Training. This is being organised by the SEM committee and there is growing interest in adding this subject into the undergraduate curriculum. The next few years will see new specialities evolving so keep your eyes open!

Already there are universities that run postgraduate MSc programmes in SEM. The Royal London Hospital, University College London and the Universities of Bath, Glasgow, Nottingham, Ulster and Wales are to name but a few and this list is likely to grow. If an MSc seems daunting then a diploma can be sat through the RCS of Edinburgh.

For further information contact the following organisations.

- UK Association of Doctors in Sport at http://www.ukadis.org/
- British Association of Sports and Exercise Medicine at http://www.basem.co.uk/index.php
- Royal College of Physicians website on the SEM committee at http://www.rcplondon.ac.uk/college/committee/sem/index.asp

## What If Medicine Is Not for You?

Some may find that, despite six or so years at medical school, when you graduate and get stuck into your pre-registration house officer (PRHO) year that a career in medicine is not for you. Firstly, this is not an uncommon feeling and there will be very few individuals who do not experience this emotion at some point, although rarely will you find your friends and colleagues expressing it openly. Secondly, it is not a disaster. I cannot emphasise this enough. Sure, you have spent a few years and a lot of money studying hard only to find out that, at the end of it, you do not like what you are doing. It is far better to discover that early on in your potential career than when you are 30 something and a registrar. Opportunities abound for qualified doctors in fields that do not involve patients. However, a word of warning: try and finish your PRHO/FY1 year at all costs, as the opportunities are far greater if you are a registered doctor and the door is left open should you wish to return. You may even change your mind.

### Research
There are always lots of research programmes going on throughout the country where posts can be created for enthusiastic young doctors. There is no specific method of obtaining a job, but word of mouth works well. Try telephoning institutes, laboratories and hospitals. Speak to consultants and heads of department. Post your CV to as many people as possible. Find a field of interest and pursue it.

### Pharmaceutical Industry
Jobs abound. Just get in touch with your local drug representative for each company (your SpR or consultant will be able to supply names and telephone numbers). Ask them to find out contact names of recruiting teams.

### Media
There is the potential for more senior doctors both to offer medical advice but also for assistance in script writing and screenplay.

## *Management*

Doctors make good managers: they are good at multi-tasking and timekeeping as well as working well under pressure. There are usually posts available within hospitals, but also look to big city businesses such as building and commerce companies. Check the classifieds in the broadsheet newspapers or your local press for job details or contact information. Secondly, the National Health Service (NHS) is crying out for hospital managers who have knowledge of medicine as a whole. The main problem is that most of the mangers in the NHS are not medically minded and have no concept of what doctors and nurses actually do. For a doctor to end up as the chief executive, well, one can dream…!

# Index

Printed in the United States
By Bookmasters